A Child's Brain

*The Impact of Advanced Research
on Cognitive and Social Behaviors*

The *Journal of Children in Contemporary Society* series:

- *Young Children in a Computerized Environment*

- *Primary Prevention for Children & Families*

- *The Puzzling Child: From Recognition to Treatment*

- *Children of Exceptional Parents*

- *Childhood Depression*

- *Newcomers to the United States: Children and Families*

- *Child Care: Emerging Legal Issues*

- *A Child's Brain: The Impact of Advanced Research on Cognitive and Social Behaviors*

- *Teachers: Economic Growth and Society*

- *Infant Intervention Programs: Truths and Untruths*

- *Marketing Child Care Programs: Why and How*

A Child's Brain

*The Impact of Advanced Research
on Cognitive and Social Behaviors*

Edited by
Mary Frank, MS in Education

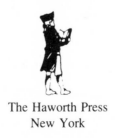

The Haworth Press
New York

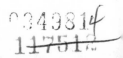

A Child's Brain: The Impact of Advanced Research on Cognitive and Social Behaviors has also been published as *Journal of Children in Contemporary Society*, Volume 16, Numbers 1/2, Fall/Winter 1983.

The Haworth Press, Inc., 28 East 22 Street, New York, NY 10010

Library of Congress Cataloging in Publication Data
Main entry under title:

A Child's brain.

Includes bibliographical references.
1. Cognition in children—Research. 2. Neuropsychology—
Research. 3. Brain—Research. 4. Child psychology—Teacher
training. I. Frank, Mary (Mary Isabelle) [DNLM: 1. Brain—Growth and development.
2. Cognition—In infancy and childhood. 3. Social behavior—In infancy and childhood.
4. Learning—In infancy and childhood.
WS 105.5.C7 F828c]
BF723.C5C515   1984   155.4′13   84-678
ISBN 0-86656-269-9

A Child's Brain

*The Impact of Advanced Research
on Cognitive and Social Behaviors*

Journal of Children in Contemporary Society
Volume 16, Numbers 1/2

CONTENTS

IMPACT ON LEARNING BEHAVIORS

FUTURE ISSUES

Preface

An interest in the brain requires no justification other than a curiosity to know why we are here, what we are doing here, and where we are going.

Paul MacLean
Director of the Laboratory
of Brain Evolution and Behavior

This issue is addressed to educators who want to capture an essence of the burgeoning fields of brain research that are specifically focusing on the child's brain. Educators have ageless questions as well as timely questions. The ageless questions are: How do we learn, acquire knowledge, process information, and what is memory? The timely questions are: what are the organizational, curricular, and instructional implications?

In ancient civilization, it was believed the liver was the repository of the soul. In later times, Aristotle believed the heart to be the central organ while the brain was a cooling system for the blood as it left the heart. Until recently, it was believed that this brain, the organ that developed cultures and built civilizations, would always remain an awesome mystery. This was true until a few decades ago when three major breakthroughs occurred that marked the beginning of a new era.

Notably, Paul MacLean from the Laboratory of Brain Evolution and Behavior at the National Institute of Mental Health began publishing his studies. For the past several years, he has been studying the evolution of the brain to learn more about the brain of present-day man. Man's lower brain is anatomically and functionally similar to that of a reptile while the mid-brain is similar to that of a mammal. The significance of this discovery is that much of our social behavior is identical to that of lower vertebrate animals. What was believed to be learned behavior is really behavior inherited through an evolutionary process.

Roger Sperry and Joseph Bogen, both neurosurgeons, won the Nobel Prize for performing many of the operations that led to their seminal findings about the hemispheric processes of the brain. From their breakthrough and continued research, it is known that man's brain is divided into two distinct hemispheres, each capable of functioning independently, each functioning in a manner different from the other, and each able to function holistically. Following this breakthrough, psychologists continue to study hemispheric characteristics as they relate to learning behaviors in the classroom setting.

Computer science which has already provided a broad-range of breakthroughs, is capable of progress almost beyond man's imagination. Initially, the development of the silicon chip gave brain researchers the tool to study the chemical, electrical, and blood transactions that occur at a split-second rate simultaneously in the brain. In addition, to better understanding the brain structure and development, the computer is being used as an assist to understand brain functions; primarily, how man processes information. The development of artificial intelligence, as fathered by Herbert Simon, a Nobel Prize winner, has provided the impetus to better understand this process.

Parenthetically, it is important for educators to recognize that the advancement of information processing is emerging from a new field called cognitive science, a science that includes the expertise of those in the neurosciences, the behavioral sciences, social sciences, and most recently, the computer sciences. The neuropsychologists and cognitive psychologists will become important adjuncts to educators.

For educators, these three breakthroughs are providing NEW BEGINNINGS. The contents of this issue are specifically designed to discuss the breakthroughs as they relate to educators as well as discuss the translation of recent brain research into practice.

In the introduction, Robert Sylwester, an educator, reviews one of the three breakthroughs, the computer. Its ability to monitor brain functions under various conditions, including learning tasks, can provide educators with new insights as to how the brain assimilates and processes information. To date, the best that educators can do with this information is to ask questions and perceive changes within the near and distant future. Sylwester proposes that it is imperative for educators to incorporate recent brain research findings into educational theory and practice.

The second section is purposefully theoretical as it provides the background for educators to understand the theory behind the known, but limited, applied practices that are discussed in the third section. From the extensive research on animals, Paul MacLean is able to trace the origins and evolution of inherent social behaviors. Timothy Teyler, a neurobiologist, wrote an in-depth article specifically geared to the ultimate concerns of educators; the role of individual neurons and specialized regions play in linguistic and higher order processing skills as well as genetic and environmental influences on brain development. The extention of Teyler's article was written by Nick Chiaia, a neurobiologist. He addresses a question of mutual concern to educators and neuroscientists, "how learning works." In summary, he discusses three major components related to processing information; the sensory and perceptual systems, the integration of information; and the output of information. He concludes with a discussion on the biological bases for cognitive and learning disorders. The proliferation of literature on hemispheric specializations, some of which is accurate and some of which is inaccurate, is brought into focus by Susan Levine, a developmental psychologist.

The third section is the section that attempts to *bridge the gap* between neuroscience and education. It is the "how-to" section. Patricia Arlin describes cognitive level matching, a method based on neurobiological research, as a process to formally and informally assess the cognitive levels of students as well as provide a system to adapt instructional material. This method is now being tested in a pilot project at the Shoreham-Wading River School in Shoreham, New York. The theory, practice, and implementation of this process is described in a companion article by Martin Brooks, Esther Fusco, and other faculty members involved in the project. Chris Pappas, who has a dual background in language studies and neurology reviews the relationship between language development and brain development specifically as it relates to oral and written language.

The development of memory skills remains as awesome and mysterious today as it did centuries ago. However, it is known that the use of specific strategies will improve memory development. Fabricius and Wellman discuss *metamemory,* a strategy used spontaneously by young children as well as other strategies that can be taught to all children. Much of what is known about the brain has been learned from war veterans suffering from head injuries as well as from head-injured children. It has been only recently that efforts to rehabilitate the head-injured child and adult have begun to receive attention. Kevin Henry describes cognitive rehabilitation therapy as the process used to rehabilitate the traumatically head-injured child along with intervention techniques used in the treatment process in a classroom setting. Harold Gordon describes the available tests that are used to assess cognitive functions of the child along with *why* the microcomputer will be used to assess normal children and children with learning disabilities.

The fourth section is the futuristic section. David Straham and Conrad Toepfer discuss the future impact of neuroscience on the education profession. They describe the emerging field of neuropsychology as offering the base for developing new learning theories, a field that includes a data base from the neurosciences, education, and developmental psychology. They advocate the implementation of this theory to all levels of education; beginning at the pre-school level and extending it through the graduate level which includes all the schools with specialized disciplines.

As was stated initially, this issue attempts to capture the ever-broadening range of research that will ultimately effect all men, women, and children in our society. This issue is best summed by Richard Restak, a neurologist, in his book *The Brain: The Last Frontier.* He wrote, "By the turn of the century, I suspect our approach to the brain will be radically different from our present orientation."

We wish to express our deep gratitude to those who created this issue. Herb Morgan, PhD, Elementary Principal, Bethlehem-Center School District, Fredericktown, PA, possesses an impressive background and understanding of this subject, and was, likewise, extremely capable of suggesting and supporting the conceptualization of this issue. The contributors, themselves, provided rich, substantive articles that reflect their own comprehensions of a complex subject. Indeed, their credibility as experts has been well earned. And there is always a significant person behind the scenes. In this case, it is Linda Cohen from The Haworth Press who originally suggested that this be a double-volume issue and whose hand gave this publication its final professional touch.

MIF

A Child's Brain

The Impact of Advanced Research
on Cognitive and Social Behaviors

INTRODUCTION

The Neurosciences and the Education Profession: Inserting New Knowledge of a Child's Developing Brain into an Already Well-Developed School

Robert Sylwester, PhD

ABSTRACT. This article (1) discusses historic technological barriers to the use of the brain in teaching/learning theory, (2) compares the medical profession's early move to biological research to the education profession's long reticence, (3) describes new brain monitoring technology that is rapidly increasing our knowledge of brain operations, and (4) proposes greater involvement of the education profession in further brain research and related technological developments.

The educational profession is at the edge of a major transformation. We have never really understood the brain that defines the teaching act, and so we tended to ignore it. However, recent dramatic developments in brain research and technology suggest that a comprehensive functional understanding of the human brain may now be within reach, and we cannot afford to ignore that developing new knowledge.

Robert Sylwester is Professor of Education, University of Oregon, Eugene, OR 97403.

The human brain is the best organized three pounds of matter in the universe, but its awesome complexity has always been a barrier to its study and understanding. For example, at the cellular level, the brain's three pint mass is divided between ten billion or more neurons (which monitor and regulate cognitive activity) and the much smaller and more numerous glial cells (which provide the support, insulation, and nourishment the neurons need to function efficiently). Further, each of these neurons is synaptically connected to thousands of other neurons in an intricate communicative network that places any neuron only a few neurons away from any other neuron in the brain's continuous flow of electrochemical transactions.

Since a space the size of a pinhead can contain more than 30,000 interconnected neurons, it is obvious that brain researchers had problems when they tried to sort out the activity of individual neurons. Studying the combined activity of aggregates of related neurons had its problems also. For example, one major connection, the 200 million nerve fiber corpus callosum that links the brain's right and left hemispheres, carries several billion bits of information every second—but it's not immediately apparent what the information is.

EDUCATORS IGNORE THE BRAIN

Brain researchers had the freedom to study patiently what they could of the brain, and wait for the development of more sophisticated chemical assay and monitoring technology to study the remainder. Our teaching profession did not have that freedom. Every fall, a new batch of students arrived at the school door, whether we understood how their brains developed and functioned or not. To carry out our professional assignment, we had to find a way to bypass the brain and its processes.

Our solution was to focus on the visible aspects of cognition. The human brain uses perceptual processes to take in objects and events from the environment. It then draws on memory and various problem-solving strategies to process this information, and it eventually translates thought and decision into behavior. If our profession could not work directly with internal brain processes, we could focus on the external objects/events in the environment (stimulus) and the behavior (response). Thus, we became a profession of behaviorists, whether we liked it or not. We learned how to manipulate the student's environment to achieve desired behavior. We did not do all that badly with this approach. Millions of intelligent sharing teachers each observing the behaviors of about thirty students for a thousand hours every year eventually learned many practical and effective things about teaching and learning. When the findings of formal educational and psychological research were added to this, our professional knowledge base increased measurably.

To be honest, though, the practical base of our profession was probably closer to folklore knowledge. We came to know what would probably occur, but we generally did not know why. Our professional folklore was replete with information such as the following: more boys than girls will have troubles in learning how to read; most hyperactive children will be boys. We knew these things, but we did not know why.

The problem with this kind of limited knowledge is that it can often lead to inappropriate conclusions at the practitioner level (e. g., that boys are stupid and ill-mannered) if all we know is from the behavior we can observe. In the end, we could never be sure whether our students learned because of our efforts, or despite them.

THE MEDICAL PROFESSION: A MESSAGE FOR EDUCATORS

For much of its history, the medical profession operated at a similar level of professional folklore. Doctors used remedies that often worked, but they did not know why they worked. The romantic vision of the pioneer family doctor is of a caring and sometimes helpful person whose diagnosis of an illness was often correct, but who also often had to sit helpless at the bedside as the patient died. The medical profession could easily handle the mild illnesses when the body's own defensive system was functioning well, but it was much less effective with illnesses that were beyond the body's own powerful recuperative powers. When the medical profession began to focus its energies on the knowledge, procedures, and technologies they needed to understand the structure and chemistry of the inside of the body and its organs, the profession's ability to diagnose and treat serious illness effectively increased tremendously. Education is now approaching a similar crossroads. We can continue to focus our energies on the careful observation of external behavior, and remain effective with teaching/learning problems that the brain can easily handle; or we can also begin to look inside the structure and chemistry of the brain for solutions to the difficult teaching/learning problems that have long plagued our profession.

A BRAIN STUDIES A BRAIN

The human brain is awesomely complex, but it is also necessarily elegantly simple. Life could not go on if the brain functioned through the random firing of billions of neurons. The key to understanding cognitive behavior lays in locating synchronized activity in aggregates of related neurons, and in discovering the factors that trigger such activity: unconscious responses, recurring rhythmic patterns, learned programmed behaviors, unique responses. Therefore, it became necessary to develop brain monitoring technology that could (1) collect vast amounts of electrochemical data from the brain, (2) summarize and interpret the significant data and ignore the rest, and (3) graphically report activity in a manner that researchers could comprehend.

The development of the silicon chip about fifteen years ago opened up this possibility. The silicon chip permitted a relatively small computer to gather and rapidly process vast amounts of data, and brain researchers seized on this technological breakthrough. Computer graphics could now take them beyond the limited two dimensional black and white EEG/X-ray reports into the world of three dimensional color TV reports.

The brain monitoring technology that evolved focuses on the overall structure of the brain, and on three aspects of neuron operation, (1) chemical transmit/inhibit decisions made within the neuron, (2) the electrical transmission of transmit decisions along the axon to other neurons, and (3) the distribution of blood through the brain as it replenishes energy used in the electrochemical transactions of cognitive activity.

Two new monitoring devices focus on the anatomical structure of the body and brain, providing a map of the location of features and disturbances. The CAT-scan (Computer-Assisted Tomography) uses multiple X-rays to provide the depth of field that simple X-rays do not provide, resulting in much clearer cross-sectional views of features. X-rays report only the shadows of structures such as bones, and pass through soft tissue. Since the brain is composed of soft tissue, the development of the NMR (Nuclear Magnetic Resonance) was a substantial step forward in brain monitoring technology. NMR responds to chemical differences in the composition of various brain/body tissues, ignores bones, and moving blood. Thus, it provides a clear picture of the chemical composition of tissue.

The EEG (Electroencephalogram) has been used for over half a century to record patterns in the electrical transmission of information within the brain. However, it was difficult to visualize brain activity from a score of squiggly lines on a moving sheet of paper, and the convolutions of the cerebral cortex made it difficult to pinpoint the source of electrical activity. Now, the recently developed BEAM (Brain Electrical Activity Mapping) machine translates the squiggly lines into various red/blue color intensities in a computer to produce on a color TV screen a much more easily understood graphic representation of the areas of positive/negative charge in the cerebral cortex. BEAM research has already disclosed patterns of brain wave activity associated with dyslexia. MEG (Magnetoencephalogram) is yet another monitoring device to improve on the EEG. It uses the magnetic fields generated by brain activity to pinpoint the location of activity much more precisely than the EEG.

PET (Positon-Emission Tomography) monitors blood distribution patterns in the brain to trace sequential changes in brain energy use, as various parts of the brain are activated in cognition. It is an exciting development because it shows the life that throbs through the house pictured by CAT and NMR.

These new brain monitoring developments supplement the parallel explosion in laboratory research made possible by new developments in brain chemistry, drug research, microscope technology, and spectrometry, and by new research procedures in psychology.

A silicon chip has helped to open the cover of the black box we call the human brain, and we can anticipate further developments that will give us an even clearer functional understanding of the micro/macro-organization and operation of the brain.

The focus of most of this research and monitoring technology has been on medical problems, and not on learning disabilities and effective teaching strategies. The medical profession has a two generation jump on us in this field, and it has a tradition of investing heavily in basic research and technology (PET machinery costs $3,000,000, and a single PET-scan costs $5000).

As the technology develops, we can anticipate that researchers will also move into areas of interest to educators, but we will need to get directly involved with the research and technology if we hope to get our problems on the research agenda.

A PROFESSION STUDIES THE BRAIN

Educators are interested in two major concerns, (1) the organizational, curricular, and instructional adaptations that brain research may suggest, and (2) the development of clear, simple, functional explanations of the brain and its complex processes that we can use to introduce our students to their own developing brain.

It would seem that almost all areas of current brain research would be of interest to educators, but some research questions seem especially significant.

- What impact do early chemical and instructional interventions have on the normal development of the brain?
- What roles do such factors as genetics, recurring rhythmic patterns, and motivation play in triggering individual cognitive activities, extended cognitive developments?
- What instructional strategies are most appropriate when dealing with learning disabilities, or rehabilitation after brain injury?
- What factors enhance memory, creativity, the mastery of skills?
- How can brain monitoring technology be adapted to the diagnostic/instructional needs of schools?
- What role might the school of the future play in developing greater conscious control over normally unconscious brain functions?

Research questions such as these will certainly be tackled and probably solved in the years ahead. Unfortunately, many in our profession today lack the scientific background to understand the research findings and implications, let alone to participate in the research, or to create curricula around it. It is a rare elementary teacher education student who takes much academic work in biology, chemistry, and cognitive psychology. Elementary teacher education students today generally major in the social sciences, and this is perhaps appropriate in light of the traditional view of teaching as a negotiated activity in a group setting.

The situation is changing. Our rapidly developing understanding of the human brain suggests that substantial changes ought to occur in our preservice and inservice teacher education programs. We will need to drastically upgrade our profession's scientific literacy.

Think back a decade and recall where brain research (or space flight, or computer technology) was then, and where it is now. Project forward a decade, and imagine what our level of understanding of the brain might be then. Can we afford not to begin the long task of reorienting our profession from its traditional focus on the normative behavior of a class group to the specific developmental needs of thirty brains?

If we continue at our current low level of knowledge of the educational aspects of the neurosciences, our profession will become vulnerable to all sorts of pseudoscientific fads, generalizations, and programs that will surely arise—consider what has already happened to the R/L hemisphere research. If teachers cannot assume informed leadership in instructional issues, they can expect that key professional decisions they ought to make will be made for them by (probably) equally uninformed administrators and lay boards. The medical profession upgraded its practitioners with solid preservice and inservice programs, and we need to seriously consider the same. Unfortunately, the rapid increase in scientific knowledge today will not give us the same extended period the medical profession had to adapt to change.

Imagine what would have happened if the medical profession had opted to stay with home remedies when it reached a similar point of decision a couple of generations ago.

FURTHER READING

Mass circulation magazines have recently published informative articles for general readers on the brain and brain monitoring research/technology. These include:

Adler, J. New looks inside the body. *Newsweek,* 1982, *8/16,* 56-69.

Begley, S. How the brain works. *Newsweek,* 1983, *2/9,* 40-47.

Buchsbaum, M. The mind readers. *Psychology Today,* 1983, *7,* 58–62.

Krassner, M. Brain Chemistry. *Chemical and Engineering News,* 1983, 8/29, 22-33.

McKean, K. Beaming new light on the brain. *Discover,* 1981, *12,* 30-33.

Sylwester, R. A child's brain. *The Instructor Magazine,* 1982, a three part series in the Sept., Oct., and Nov. issues.

Wright, S. Cerebral scanners, *Equinox,* 1982, *7,* 42-55.

Zimmerman, J. MEG gets inside your head. *Psychology Today,* 1982, *4,* 100.

BRAIN STRUCTURE

Brain Evolution: The Origins of Social and Cognitive Behaviors

Paul MacLean, MD

ABSTRACT. This article is a compilation of three articles written by Paul MacLean (refer to Footnote). Based on his research, MacLean states that there are common anatomical and functional characteristics among the brains of reptiles, mammals, and man. For educators, the most significant commonality is that of social behavior. Frequently, behaviors that are observed in the classroom, and believed to be learned, are actually inherited through the evolutionary process. To describe and illustrate this phenomenon, MacLean places it in the context of a model he terms the "triune brain": the reptilian, the paleomammalian, and the neomammalian brain.

INTRODUCTION

Many people point out the apparent irony that the great strides in the natural sciences seem to be speeding us toward the Hill of Megiddo and the long-advertised final conflict between the forces of good and evil. Others, still blinded by the searing light of Hiroshima, are more introspective in expressing this concern: How, they ask, can we contain and harness the devastating powers of the atom before we have learned to understand and control the potentially catastrophic forces within ourselves?

Paul MacLean, is Chief, Laboratory of Brain Evolution and Behavior, National Institute of Mental Health, Poolesville, MD 20837.

9

In recent years anxiety about thermonuclear war has diminished somewhat in the light of warnings that the human race and many forms of life may be on the way to extinction because of scientific developments that have made possible overpopulation, pollution of the environment, and exhaustion of critical resources.

A curve showing the growth of the world's population (Foerster, Mora, & Amiot, 1960) indicates that each successive doubling of people has taken place in half the time of the previous doubling (Calhoun, 1971). At this rate the present population would be expected to double in 30 or 40 years. In 1969, U Thant, speaking as Secretary of the United Nations, made his famous pronouncement that there remained only 10 years to find solutions for the exploding population and related problems.

Warnings of this kind focus attention almost exclusively on the external environment. It is so easy to see the problems of meeting future demands for food, water, energy, and other basic requisites that planning experts seem to have overlooked the lessons of animal experimentation indicating that psychological "stresses" of crowding may bring about a collapse of social structure despite an ample provision of the necessities of life (Calhoun, 1962; Myers, Hale, Myktowycz, & Hughes, 1971). Systems analysts who have attempted to predict the limits of growth with the aid of computer technology (Meadows, D. H., Meadows, D. L., Randers & Behrens, 1972) either admit to an inability to deal with psychological factors or neglect them altogether.

Michael Chance (1969) has remarked that the parts of the universe that man first chose for study were those furthest removed from the self—meaning, of course, the heavens and the science of astronomy. By contrast, and perhaps for similar reasons, there has been a retarded interest in turning the dissecting lamp of the scientific method onto the inner self and the psychological instrument by which we derive all scientific knowledge. It would almost seem that there had always been a supernatural injunction against doing so.

SYNOPSIS OF EXPERIMENTAL WORK

For the past 25 years, my research has been primarily concerned with identifying and analyzing forebrain mechanisms underlying prosematic (nonverbal language) forms of behavior which on phylogenetic and clinical grounds might be inferred to represent expressions of "paleopsychic" processes. In this work, I have taken a comparative evolutionary approach which has the advantage that it allows one to telescope millions of years into a span that can be seen all at once, and as in plotting a curve makes it possible to see trends that would not otherwise be apparent. It also shows the usefulness of research on animals for obtaining insights into brain mechanisms underlying human prosematic behavior.

Since animal experimentation provides us our only systematic knowledge of brain functions, I should comment briefly on the justification of using findings on animals for drawing inferences about the workings of the human brain. At the molecular or cellular levels, there is general enthusiasm for applying findings on animals to human biology. Many people believe that behavioral and neurological observations on animals have little or no human relevance.

Such a bias perhaps stems from a failure to realize that in its evolution, the human brain expands in hierarchic fashion along the lines of three basic patterns (Figure 1) as reptilian, paleomammalian (old brain), and neomammalian (new brain). The three formations are markedly different in chemistry and structure and in an evolutionary sense are eons apart. Extensively interconnected, the three basic formations represent an amalgamation of three-brains-in-one, on what may be appropriately called *a triune* brain (MacLean, 1970, 1973 (a), 1973 (b)). The word triune also serves to imply that the "whole" is greater than the sum of its parts, because with the exchange of information among the three formations each derives a greater amount of information than if it were operating alone. Stated in popular terms, the amalgamation amounts to three interconnected biological computers, with each inferred to have its own special intelligence, its own subjectivity, its own sense of time and space, and its own memory, motor, and other functions.

This scheme for subdividing the brain may seem simplistic, but thanks to improved neuro anatomical, physiological, and chemical techniques, the three basic formations stand out in clearer detail than ever before. Moreover, it should be emphasized that despite their extensive interconnections, there is evidence that each brain type is capable of operating somewhat independently. Most important in regard to the "verbal-nonverbal" question, there are clinical indications that the reptilian and paleomammalian formations lack the neural machinery for verbal communication. To say that they lack the power of speech, however, does not belittle their intelli-

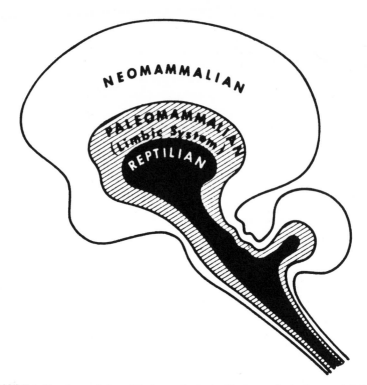

FIGURE 1. Showing evolution of the human forebrain. The human forebrain expands in hierarchic fashion along the lines of three basic patterns that may be characterized as reptilian, paleomammalian, and neomammalian.

SOURCE: Paul D. MacLean, "The Brain in Relation to Empathy and Medical Education," *Journal of Nervous and Mental Disease* 144 (1967): 374-82.

gence, nor does it relegate them subjectively to the realm of the "unconscious."

The basic neural machinery required for self-preservation and the preservation of the species is built into the neural chassis contained in the midbrain, pons, medulla, and spinal cord. As shown by the early experiments of Farrier (1876) and others, an animal with only its neural chassis is as motionless and aimless as an idling vehicle without a driver. But this analogy stops short because with the evolution of the forebrain, the neural chassis acquires three drivers, all of different minds and all vying for control.

THE REPTILIAN-TYPE BRAIN

Let us look first at the reptilian "driver." In mammals, the major counterpart of the reptilian forebrain is represented by a group of large ganglia including the olfactostriatum, corpus striatum, globus pallidus, and satellite gray matter. Since there is no name that applies to all of these structures, I shall refer to them as the R-Complex. Lizards and other reptiles provide illustrations of complex prototypical *patterns* of behavior commonly seen in mammals, including man. One can quickly list more than 20 such behaviors that may primarily involve self-preservation or the survival of the species (MacLean, 1974): (1) selection and preparation of homesite, (2) establishment of domain or territory, (3) tail making, (4) "marking" of domain or territory, (5) showing place-preferences, (6) ritualistic display in defense of territory, commonly involving the use of coloration and adornment, (7) formalized intraspecific fighting in defense of territory, (8) triumphal display in successful defense, (9) assumption of distinctive postures and coloration in signalling surrender, (10) routinization of daily activities, (11) foraging, (12) hunting, (13) homing, (14) hoarding, (15) use of defecation posts, (16) formation of social groups, (17) establishment of social hierarchy by ritualistic display and other means, (18) greeting, (19) "grooming," (20) courtships, with displays using coloration and adornments, (21) mating, (22) breeding and, in isolated instances, attending offspring, (23) flocking. Except for altruistic behavior and most aspects of parental behavior, it is remarkable how many *patterns of behavior* seen in reptiles are also found in human beings.

THE PALEOMAMMALIAN BRAIN

There are behavioral indications that the reptilian brain is poorly equipped for learning to cope with new situations. The reptilian brain has only a rudimentary cortex. In the lost transitional forms between reptiles and mammals—the so-called mammal-like reptiles—it is presumed that the primitive cortex underwent further elaboration and differentiation. The primitive cortex might be imagined as comparable to a rude radar screen, providing the animal a better means of viewing the environment and learning to survive. In all existing mammals the phylogenetically old cortex is found in a large convolution which the nineteenth century anatomist, Broca (1878) called the great limbic lobe because it surrounds the brain stem. Limbic means "forming a border around." The limbic lobe forms a *common denominator* in the brains of *all mammals*. In 1952, I suggested the term limbic system as a designation for the limbic cortex and structures of the brain stem with which it has primary connections (MacLean, 1952).

The limbic cortex is structurally less complicated than the new cortex. Although it was once believed to receive information mainly from the olfactory and visceral systems, we have shown by recording from single nerve cells in awake, sitting monkeys that signals also reach it from the visual, auditory, and somatic senses (MacLean, 1973b). There are clinical indications that the combined reception of information from the inside and outside worlds is essential for a feeling of individuality and personal identity (MacLean, 1972).

Also in contrast to the new cortex, the limbic cortex has large cablelike connections with the hypothalamus which has long been recognized to play a central role in integrating the performance of mechanisms involved in self-preservation and the procreation of the species.

Although the limbic system undergoes considerable expansion in the brains of higher mammals, the basic pattern of organization remains the same as in lower mammals. Electrophysiological studies have shown that this basically paleomammalian brain is functionally, as well as anatomically, an integrated system. In the past 40 years, clinical and experimental investigations have provided evidence that the limbic system derives information in terms of emotional feelings that guide behavior with respect to the two basic life principles of self-preservation and the preservation of the species.

Before further comment on limbic functions, it should be noted that many people maintain that it is inadmissible to make sharp distinction between "emotion" and "reason." Raphael Demos (1937), in an introduction to the dialogues of Plato, expresses a traditional philosophical view: ". . . we are apt to separate reason from emotion. Plato does not. Reason is not merely detached understanding; it is conviction, fired with enthusiasm." Piaget, the founder of the Center for Genetic Epistemology, is quite vehement, saying that "nothing could be more false or superficial" than to attempt "to dichotomize the life of the mind into emotion and thoughts." ". . . Affectivity and intelligence," he insists, "are indissociable and constitute the two complementary aspects of all human behavior" (Piaget, 1967, p. 15).

Three Subdivisions of the Paleomammalian Brain

The limbic system comprises three subdivisions (MacLean, 1958). The two older ones are closely related to the olfactory apparatus. Our experimental work has provided evidence that these two divisions are involved respectively in oral and genital functions. The findings are relevant to orosexual manifestations in feeding situations, in mating, and in aggressive behavior and violence. The close relationship between oral and genital functions seems to be due to the olfactory sense which, dating far back in evolution, is involved in both feeding and mating.

The main pathway to the third subdivision bypasses the olfactory apparatus. In evolution, this subdivision reaches its greatest development in the human brain. An assortment of evidence suggests that this remarkable expansion reflects a shift from olfactory to visual and other influences in sociosexual behavior. It is also possible that this subdivision, together with the prefrontal cortex of the neomammalian brain, has provided a neural substrate for the evolution of human empathy.

Avenues to the Basic Personality

The major pathways to and from the reptilian-type and paleomammalian-type brains pass through the hypothalamus and subthalamic region (Figure 2). If the majority of these pathways are destroyed in monkeys, they are greatly incapacitated, but with careful nursing may recover the ability to feed themselves and move around. The most striking characteristic of these animals is that although they look like monkeys, they no longer behave like monkeys. Almost everything characteristic of species-typical simian behavior has disappeared. If one were to interpret these experimental findings in the light of certain clinical case material, one might say that these large connecting pathways between the reptilian and paleomammalian formations provide the avenues to the basic personality. Here, certainly, would seem to be the pathways to the expression of prosematic behavior.

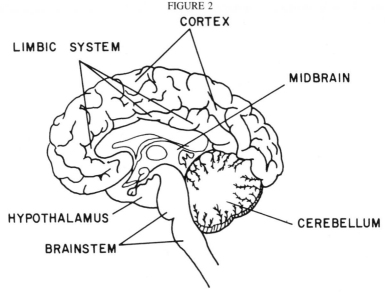

FIGURE 2

Illustration courtesy of Timothy Teyler.

THE NEOMAMMALIAN BRAIN

To credit the two older evolutionary formations of the psychencephalon with providing the underpinnings of basic behavior is not to downplay the importance of the neocortex. As for human beings, nothing is more neurologically certain than that the neocortex provides the neural substrate for language and speech and that we owe to it the infinite variety of ways in which we can express ourselves. The neocortex mushrooms progressively in high mammals and reaches its greatest development in human beings.

Compared with the limbic cortex, the neocortex is like an expanding numerator. As C. Judson Herrick (1933) has commented, "Its explosive growth late in phylogeny is one of the most dramatic cases of evolutionary transformations known to comparative anatomy." The massive proportions achieved by the neocortex in higher mammals explains the designation of "neomammalian brain" applied to it and structures of the brain stem with which it is primarily connected. The neocortex culminates in the human brain, affording a vast neural screen for the portrayal of symbolic language and the associated functions of reading, writing, and arithmetic. Mother of invention and father of abstract thought, it promotes the preservation and precreation of ideas (MacLean, 1973a). As opposed to the limbic cortex, the sensory systems projecting to the neocortex are primarily those giving information about the external environment—namely, the visual, auditory, and somatic systems. It therefore seems that the neocortex is primarily oriented toward the outside world.

Handedness and Speech

Lack of available space prevents discussion of the protean functions identified with neocortical systems. From the standpoint of primate evolution, it would be particularly pertinent to consider the factors that have accounted for the tie-in of vocalization with handedness and speech. This subject, however, invariably ends up on the shoals of speculation. Take, for example, the question as to why most human beings are right-handed—a condition that, according to artifacts of prehistory, has existed for thousands of years (Coren & Porac, 1977). As a caveat in regard to the complexity of the problem, a predisposition to "rightness" in some form exists among some snails, flatfish, and other animals. Elsewhere I have speculated about the evolution of handedness (MacLean, 1978b), starting with Thomas Carlyle's "primitive warfare theory" and giving it a new twist in connection with Raymond Dart's osteodontokeratic Culture (1959). Given the inherited predisposition to right-handedness, one can develop an explanation of the cerebral dominance of speech, first noting how it would be neurologically advantageous for a midline organ of speech such as the tongue with its bilateral innervation to receive its commands from a single hemisphere (MacLean, 1978b). The representation of speech in the left hemisphere would provide the quickest and most effective means of coordinating speech and right-handed action. It is evident how under conditions of group hunting or of internecine strife, split-second timing in enunciating a directional signal might make the difference between life and death.

The same neurological economy with respect to dominance would apply to a written language, because whenever the idea first struck to jot things down, the right hand was ready and waiting!

That the nondominant hemisphere sits idly by without ever mastering a language has been considered a great functional waste. In the light of computer technology, I suggested that this seeming deficiency may have compensations. With computers, an insufficient "memory" presents a continuing hindrance to achieving solutions of complicated problems. One might propose that nature, in placing linguistic functions in one hemisphere, killed two birds with one stone—putting the midline organ, the tongue, under a single command and freeing the nondominant hemisphere to be used for a greatly expanded memory (MacLean, 1978b). There is evidence that the nondominant hemisphere plays a role in the registration of memories (Penfield & Milner, 1958; Milner, Corkin, & Teuber, 1968).

Transcendent Speech

In an evolutionary sense, the "isolation call" is probably the oldest and most basic of mammalian vocalizations, serving to maintain maternal-offspring contact, as well as contact with other members of the same species. In squirrel monkeys we found that gray matter at the core of the forebrain (posterior periventricular gray) appears to be essential for the production of these calls (Newman & MacLean, 1981). This gray matter receives part of its connections from the limbic cortex. Interestingly, in view of the questioned ability of vocalization in reptiles ancestral to mammals, when the subhuman mammalian telencephalon is electrically stimulated, vocalization can be elicited only from limbic structures (Jurgens & Ploog, 1970). The vocalization required for speech appears to have necessitated a quantum jump to the neocortex. Electrical stimulation of the so-called speech areas interferes with our speech, but does not produce speech (Penfield & Jasper, 1954).

Curiously, the human brain attained its large size thousands of years before there was a language of words. And just as curiously, it has been only two thousand years since human beings first saw the "sunya" (the empty space, the "zero," existing between the fingers) that has since afforded a workable language of numbers (Hogben, 1937). With the soaring developments in modern communication, who is to say what other languages, what metalanguages, what transcendent speech, may still be in the making?

That one form of transcendent speech is in the making, we may be quite sure. As though an essential ingredient had been left out, a new sector of cortex appears in the neomammalian brain that ties in with interoceptive systems. This relatively recent neocortical development turns our attention once more to mammalian evolution and the evolution of the human family. The location of the cortical development in question becomes apparent by contrasting the low brow of a Neanderthal skull and the recently evolved high brow of a Cro-Magnon skull. Underneath the high brow is a greatly expanded sector of cortex that appears to be the only neocortex that establishes a strong communicative link with the internal world.

Time and Space

Although nuclear physicists are quick to point out the "evaporation" of the material world at the atomic level, many of them seem to retain an abiding faith in the existence of time and space. They would contend that if all particles were to disappear from the universe, space and time would still remain. There is an evident inconsistency in such an argument when we relook at what Kant said about the "transcendental aesthetic." In view of the tripartite division of the brain under consideration, we want to keep in mind the question whether there exist "reptilian time," "paleomammalian time," and "neomammalian time." A parallel question applies to space. Recently, students of environmental design have begun to consider the latter question in connection with urban planning and the desirable uses of space (Easer, 1974; Greenbie, in press; Mallows, 1970).

CONCLUDING COMMENT

I have used the expression *triune brain* to symbolize that no hard and fast boundaries exist between the three formations and their respective functions. With these provision, I use a metaphor to summarize.

In the field of literature it is recognized that there is an irreducible number of basic plots and associated emotions. In describing the functions of the triune brain metaphorically, one might imagine that the reptilian brain provides the basic plots and actions; that the limbic brain influences emotionally the developments of the plots;

while the neomammalian brain has the capacity to expound the plots and emotions in as many ways as there are authors.

FOOTNOTES

MacLean, P. On the evolution of three mentalities. In S. Arieti & G. Chrzanowski (Eds.), New dimension in psychiatry: A World View (Vol. 2). New York: John Wiley & Sons, Inc., 1977.

MacLean, P. On the origin and progressive evolution of the triune brain. In E. Armstrong & D. Falk (Eds.), Primate brain evolution: Methods and concepts. New York: Plenum Publishing Corp., 1982.

MacLean, P. The triune brain. Reprinted by the U. S. Department of Health, Education, and Welfare, National Institutes of Health.

The above articles belong to the public domain and are not subject to copyright laws.

REFERENCES

Broca, P. Anatomie comparee des circonvolutions cerebrales. Le grand lobre limbique et la scissure limbique dans la serie des mammiferes. Rev. Anthropol, 1878, 1, 385-498.

Calhoun, J. B. Population density and social pathology. Science American, 1962, 206, 139-146.

Chance, M. Towards the biological definition of ethics. In J. Ebbling (Ed.), Biology and Ethics. New York: Academic Press, 1969.

Coren, S., & Porac, C. Fifty centuries of right-handedness: The historical record. Science, 1977, 198, 631-632.

Dart, R. A. Adventures with the missing link. Philadelphia: The Institutes Press, The Institutes for the Achievement of Human Potential, 1959.

Esser, A. H. Environment and mental health. Science Medical Manual, 1974, 1, 181-193.

Ferrier, D. The Functions of the brain. London: Smith, Elder, and Company, 1876.

Foerster, H., Mora, P., & Amiot, L. Doomsday: Friday, 13 November, A. D. 2026. Science, 1960, 132, 1291-1295.

Greenbie, B. Design for Diversity. Amsterdam: Elsevier Scientific Publishing Company, in press.

Herrick, C. J. The functions of the olfactory parts of the cerebral cortex. Proc. Nat. Acad. Sci. USA, 133, 19, 7-14.

Herrick, C. J. The brain of the tiger salamander. Chicago: University of Chicago Press, 1948.

Hogben, L. Mathematics for the million. New York: W. W. Norton and Co. 1937.

Jurgens, U., & Ploog, D. Cerebral representation of vocalization in the squirrel monkey. Exp. Brain Res., 1970, 10, 532-554.

MacLean, P. Some psychiatric implications of physiological studies on frontotemporal portion of limbic system (visceral brain). Electroenceph. Clin. Neurophysiol., 1952, 4, 407-418.

MacLean, P. Contrasting functions of limbic and neocortical systems of the brain and their relevance to psychophysiological aspects of medicine. Amer. J. Med., 1958, 146, 950-952.

MacLean, P. New findings relevant to the evolution of psychosexual functions of the brain. J. Nerv. Ment. Dis., 1962, 135, 289-301.

MacLean, P. The triune brain, emotion, and scientific bias. In F. O. Schmitt (Ed.), *The neurosciences second study program*. New York: The Rockefeller University Press, 1970, pp. 336-349.

MacLean, P. Implications of microelectrode findings on exteroceptive inputs to the limbic cortes. In C. H. Hockman (ed.), *Limbic system* mechanisms and autonomic function. Springfield: Charles C Thomas, 1972, pp. 115-136.

MacLean, P. The brain's generation gap: Some human implications. *Zygon J. Relig. Sci.*, 1973(a), *8*, 113-127.

MacLean, P. A triune concept of the brain and behavior, Lecture I. Man's reptilian and limbic inheritance, Lecture II. Man's limbic brain and the psychoses, Lecture III. New trends in man's evolution. In T. Boag & D. Campbell (Eds.), *The Hincks memorial lectures*. Toronto: University of Toronto Press, 1973(b), pp. 6-66.

MacLean, P. An evolutionary approach to brain research on "prosematic" (nonverbal) behavior. In *The Daniel S. Lehrman Memorial Symposium on Reproductive Behavior and Evolution*, Institute of Animal Behavior, Rutgers University, 1974 (to be published).

MacLean, P. *A mind of three minds: Educating the triune brain.* Seventy-fifth Yearbook of the National Society for the Study of Education. Chicago: University of Chicago Press, 1978, pp. 308-342.

Mallows, E. Urban planning and the systems approach (IBM System & Engineering Symposium, October, 1969). *Plan* (Successor to S. A. Archit. Rec.), 1970, *55*, 11-24.

Meadows, D. H., Meadows, D. L., Randers, J., & Behrens, III, W. *The limits to growth.* New York: Universe Books, 1972.

Milner, B., Corkin, S., & Teuber, H. Further analysis of the hippocampal amnesic syndrome: 14-year follow-up study of H.M. *Neuropsychologia*, 1968, *6*, 215-234.

Myers, K., Hale, C., Myktowycz, R., & Hughes, R. The effects of varying density and space on sociality and health in animals. In A. H. Esser (Ed.). New York: Plenum Press, 1971, 148-187.

Newman, J., & MacLean, P. Effects of tegmental lesions on the isolation call of squirrel monkeys. *Brain Res.*, in press.

Penfield, W., & Jasper, H. *Epilepsy and the functional anatomy of the human brain.* Boston: Little, Brown, and Co., 1954.

Penfield, W., & Milner, B. Memory deficit produced by bilateral lesions in the hippocampal zone. *AMA Arch. Neurol. Psychiat.*, 1958, *79*, 475-497.

Piaget, J. *Six Psychological Studies,* Transl. A. Tenzer. New York: Random House, 1967.

Brain Structure and Development

T. J. Teyler, PhD
N. Chiaia, MA

ABSTRACT. The human brain is composed of billions of neurons. In this chapter we will examine the properties of the neuron, how neurons interact and how they are organized into subdivisions within the brain. Such information is essential as a framework that can be applied to further considerations of the brain processes involved in the more complicated behaviors of concern to educators.

INTRODUCTION

In this chapter and the one that follows, we shall be dealing with the biology and function of the brain. We realize that the readership of this journal will not have an extensive background in the neurosciences and we will attempt to refrain from using the specialized jargon of the neurosciences. In this chapter, we shall consider the basic biology of the brain, what we know of how it operates, and something of how it develops. In the next chapter, we shall consider some aspects of the ultimate expression of brain activity, that is, of course, behavior. In particular, we shall concentrate on those behaviors, and the brain processes that are most relevant to the concerns and needs of the classroom educator.

The human brain, like other brains, is composed of individual neurons. Neurobiologists have provided us with a wealth of information concerning the anatomy, physiology, and chemistry of the neuron. They are well on their way to understanding how a single neuron works, and how a few interconnected neurons operate. For those interested in more practical matters, such as educators, this wealth of information is often of little direct relevance. It is assumed, however, that the basic studies that neurobiologists are currently undertaking will eventually shed light on the brain pro-

T. J. Teyler and N. Chiaia are affiliated with the Neurobiology Program, Northeastern Ohio Universities College of Medicine, Rootstown, OH 44272.

cesses underlying higher mental operations. Currently however, the brain processes underlying higher mental operations are largely unknown. As a consequence the two disciplines of Education and Neuroscience are rather far apart. It is our goal to begin to bridge this chasm by encouraging a dialog between educators and neuroscientists. We feel that educators have much to gain by learning more about the organ they devote their careers toward shaping.

The brain mechanisms that have been studied with relation to higher mental operations and language are relatively crude. At this stage, neuroscientists have studied the brain by removing rather substantial portions of the animal brain, through the effects of human illness and accidents, and observing the effect on subsequent behavior. More recently, studies of the electrical activity of the human brain have been correlated with language function and other higher operations. These electrical recordings of brain activity, since they are done in human beings, are non-invasive, that is, they do not involve placing electrodes within the tissue of the brain, but rather involve recording the electrical activity of the brain from the surface of the scalp. Such recordings detect the activity of millions of neurons operating more or less simultaneously. In contrast, the work of many neurobiologists involves, in large part, recording the activity of single neurons, in many cases with electrodes that penetrate into the interior of the cell. Obviously such studies will never be done on normal human beings to study their brain correlates of language and higher function.

However, since the brain is composed of individual neurons, and since specialized regions of the brain can be identified, and their function described, and since this information will eventually have a bearing on the understanding of linguistic and higher order processing in the central nervous system, it is necessary to spend some time reviewing the basic structure and function of the neuron.

The Neuron

There are about 200 billion neurons in the human brain; a number so large as to be nearly meaningless. They are dwarfed only by the number of interconnections between those neurons, a figure truly astronomical. Neurons (Figure 1) are cells specialized to communicate with each other and to receive information from the outside world and to issue commands to the muscles and glands.

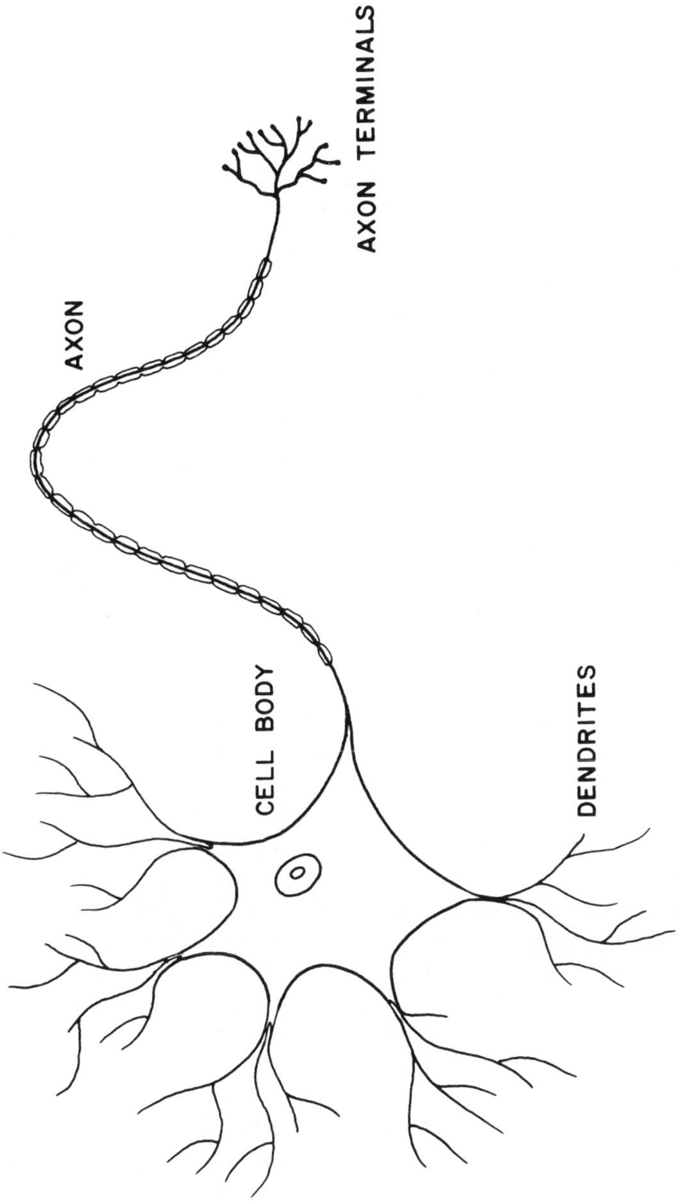

AXON

AXON TERMINALS

CELL BODY

DENDRITES

FIGURE 1

Neurons communicate with one another by secreting chemical substances called *neurotransmitters* from the ends of processes called *axons*. The axons of neurons typically extend for quite a distance from the cell body itself and typically influence thousands of other neurons.

Neuroscientists are generally not very poetic, but in describing one aspect of the neuron, they have achieved a certain degree of eloquence. The structure of the *dendritic tree* of a neuron quite closely resembles that of a botanical tree. It is upon the dendrites that the axons of other neurons release their chemical neurotransmitters. At these sites of communication, called *synapses* (from the Greek word which means to clasp or to join) the recipient cell responds to the chemicals released by the transmitting cell. Its response is possible because it possesses specialized proteins on the surface of the recipient cell. These specialized proteins, termed membrane *receptors* and found in the region of the synapse, chemically bind to the neurotransmitter chemical and effect some change in the recipient neuron.

The membrane receptors that we are discussing are located at the synaptic connection between the axon of one neuron and the dendrite of another. There are, other membrane receptors that sense the environment of the neuron. These receptors act much like endocrine glands, responding to molecules in the environment of the neuron. The concept of the receptor is a critical and central one in neurobiology (as well as in most of the rest of physiology). This is so because the surface of neurons and other cells are peppered with thousands of different kinds of receptors, each specialized for binding to particular molecules and each responsible for eliciting particular effects from the recipient cell.

The importance of membrane receptors is quite apparent in medicine and also in drug abuse. It is the interaction of drugs and medicine with membrane receptors that determines the effectiveness of many medicines and provides the pleasurable effects associated with drugs. For example, the membrane receptor for the brain neurotransmitter enkephalin also binds to the narcotic heroin, a molecule normally not present in the brain. Thus, heroin along with enkephalin, which is thought to be involved in pain sensations, have an analgesic effect. The euphoria associated with heroin usage can be attributed to the affects of these drugs on still other receptors in the brain.

In general, whenever a drug has a psychoactive effect, it is because it is interacting with membrane receptors whose normal function is being altered by the drug. One danger in utilizing any drugs that "fool" the brain into thinking that it is a neurotransmitter, is that the biochemical machinery necessary to produce the neurotransmitter may shut down. This occurs because of feedback mechanisms that shut the machinery down when there is sufficient neurotransmitter being produced. The feedback control is being "tricked" by the drug masquerading as a neurotransmitter. If the drug is not taken, the brain's biochemical machinery has shut down and is unable to produce the real neurotransmitter for a time, leading to the severe symptoms known as drug withdrawal.

To provide other concrete examples, the neurotransmitter acetylcholine is released by axons and acts upon membrane receptors located at the dendritic synapse and at nerve-muscle synapses. On the other hand, norepinephrine is released into the general vicinity of the neuron to there act upon nonsynaptic receptors of nearby neurons. The two actions are quite different; the first being limited to the recipient cell, whereas the second is more widespread and diffuse. Functionally, these differences are reflected in the quite specific effect of acetylcholine upon muscle fibers causing them to contract as opposed to the more widespread effect of norepinephrine on brain activity.

The Synapse. Dendrites are many and often very finely branched. Extending from the surface of the dendrite on many neurons are multiple, small protuberances termed *dendritic spines* (Figure 2). It is upon these dendritic spines that synaptic contacts are made from other neurons. The majority of synaptic contacts in the vertebrate utilize chemical synapses. In the chemical synapse, the axon terminal of one neuron does not physically touch the dendritic spine of another neuron, rather a tiny gap exists between these two processes. This gap is referred to as the synaptic gap.

A typical neuron in the outer covering, or cortex, of the brain may have as many as 10,000 synaptic contacts made upon it. Similarly, the axon from a particular neuron is often found to branch, thus giving rise to the possibility of a single axon making synaptic contact on to the dendrites of many thousands of neurons. One can see that with billions of neurons, each one of which has thousands of inputs and hundreds or thousands of outputs, the total number of interconnections in the human brain is indeed astronomical. It has been estimated that the number of possible interconnections between the cells in a single human brain is greater than the num-

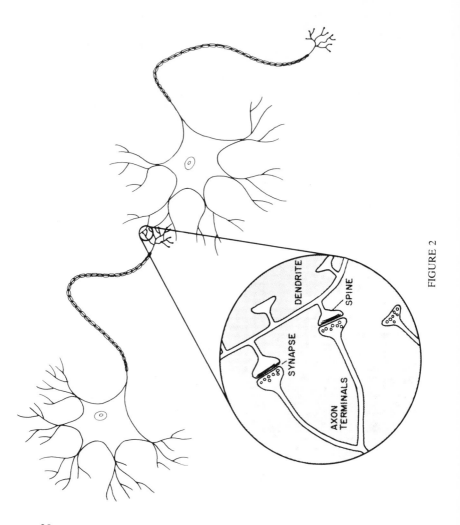

DENDRITE

SPINE

SYNAPSE

AXON
TERMINALS

FIGURE 2

ber of atoms in the known universe. While this may be somewhat of an overstatement (particularly since there may be no bounds on the universe) it does illustrate the staggering number of interconnections contained within a single human brain.

Synaptic Activity

There are two basic kinds of effects as a result of synaptic activity, one is to excite the recipient cell, whereas the other is to inhibit the cell. Each is dependent upon specific neurotransmitters. When active, a neuron generates an *action potential,* which is a rearrangement of its membrane to allow ions to flow across it, the details of which we shall not consider here.

An action potential is a wave of excitation that travels down the axon, causing neurotransmitters to be released when it reaches the end. A neuron releases its neurotransmitter when it becomes activated as a result of receiving impulses from other neurons. The activity of the nervous system, considered at this level, consists of the interplay of excitatory and inhibitory neurotransmitters converging upon the dendrites of billions of cells in the brain. Added to this is the modulating role of nonsynaptic receptors mentioned earlier.

Most neurons contain both excitatory and inhibitory synaptic inputs. At any given time both of these types of synaptic inputs may be active but to various degrees. It is the function of the neuron to integrate inhibition and excitation over the surface of the dendrites. A neuron will be made to fire by increasing the excitatory input relative to the inhibitory input. This can be done in two ways. Starting with a constant level of excitatory and inhibitory input one can cause a neuron to fire by (a) increasing the excitatory input, or by (b) decreasing the inhibitory input. Merely increasing both excitatory and inhibitory inputs will have little effect on the neurons' ability to generate an action potential. These are two of the simpler forms of neuronal integration that many neurons are capable of performing.

In the brain, neurons are usually found in functional groups. In the next section, we shall provide a thumbnail sketch of these fundamental components of the brain which considers both the structure and function.

BRAIN STRUCTURE

Components of the Brain

The basic plan of the brain was laid down eons ago and is represented today in such noble creatures as the lowly earthworm. It consists of three divisions: sensory, central processing, and motor.

Sensory Processing

In the human brain, sensory processing includes, of course, all of the specialized sensory receptors such as those located in the retina of the eye, in the cochlea of the ear, and in the surface of the skin. Also included with the sensory system are brain structures devoted to the decoding of sensory information. In the brain, the major sensory structures are the thalamus, which is a major processing center for all kinds of sensory information; and the cortical sensory areas.

Motor Processing

Skipping to the motor side of the central nervous system, we find that in the human brain, most of the neurons that control the musculature of the body are located in the spinal cord, those that control the musculature of the head and neck are located in the base of the brain. These neurons, in turn, receive their commands from other neurons higher up in the brain and constitute information of two sorts: direct information and indirect information. While the details of the anatomy of the system are much too complex to be treated here, suffice it to say that we know a good deal about the neurobiology of the motor system and can now begin to appreciate some of the medical difficulties encountered with conditions such as Parkinson's Disease.

Central Processing

While we know the most about the sensory systems and motor systems, we know the least about the central processing capabilities of the human brain. Yet, in the human, neurons devoted to the processing capabilities make up the vast bulk, probably 80-90%, of the neurons in the human brain. These neurons are devoted to information processing and are not strictly sensory or motor in function. It is these cells that are of most concern to the educator because they determine the cognitive and linguistic capabilities of the student. They determine the motivational and emotional state of students, and they determine the ability to learn and remember events over time. In the chapter on Higher Brain Function, we shall consider some of the brain circuits involved in some of the higher order operations of the brain.

Neurons that make up the central nervous system (CNS) are organized into functional groupings. For convenience and simplicity we have divided these groupings into several major categories. We will start at the simplest level of brain organization, that is, the spinal cord, and gradually work our way up to the cerebral cortex. Later in this chapter the reader will encounter such brain structures as the limbic system, the thalamus, the reticular formation, brain stem, and of course the neocortex. It is not our intention to review all of neuroanatomy in this section, rather, we wish to provide a framework that can be applied to further discussion of brain components introduced at a later point.

Neural tube. Embryonically, the central nervous system develops from a primitive neural tube. The basic structure of the embryonic brain is a sheet of neurons enclosing a central canal. This basic aspect of brain organization is preserved through CNS development such that in the adult brain one can discern a central canal filled with cerebrospinal fluid.

In the process of development this simple geometric organization of a canal surrounded by tissue becomes greatly modified. However, in the spinal cord the basic organization is still clearly evident. Therefore, we see in the spinal cord of man and other vertebrates a central canal filled with cerebrospinal fluid surrounded by cell bodies. The cell bodies are in turn surrounded by nerve tracts which are: (a) ascending into the brain, (b) descending from the brain, and (c) communicating with the periphery.

Within the cell body region of the spinal cord (the grey matter) one finds two kinds of neurons. One variety, termed principal cells, are predominately motor neurons whose axons project to the muscles of the body. These neurons are the cells that directly control the body musculature. Motor neurons receive their inputs from the nerve tracts of the spinal cord, from sensory cells whose cell bodies are located just adjacent to the spinal cord, and from local circuit neurons. The second variety, local circuit neurons, have a limited dendritic and axonal field, such that they influence principle neurons and other local circuit neurons within a very circumscribed region. These two basic neuron types found in the spinal cord are present in the brain as well and function as sensory neurons, local circuit neurons, and motor neurons.

The spinal cord is concerned with motor control, reflex activity, and the first stages of processing of sensory information from the body surface, muscles and joints. This information, in addition to being processed locally in reflexes, ascends up to the brain via long nerve tracts. The local circuit neurons in the spinal cord contribute to motor and sensory processing, and facilitate reflexive behavior.

Brain Stem. As one proceeds "up stream" into the brain we are confronted with a portion of the brain that, like the spinal cord, has changed little across evolutionary history. This area is the brain stem (Figure 3). Now we must introduce the term nucleus (plural nuclei). A nucleus is an anatomically distinct collection of neurons that generally subserve similar function. For example, in the brain stem there are nuclei of the autonomic nervous system, a relatively involuntary division of the central nervous system, that is concerned with the regulation of bodily functions and other aspects of physiologic control of which we have little conscious awareness. There are in the brain stem many nuclei concerned with sensory and motor functions and many of these nuclei relay their information to higher centers in the nervous system. Looking across phylogeny one finds that this region of the brain has changed little across a wide range of species.

Hypothalamus. As we ascend further into the brain, we come to an important structure, the hypothalamus. The hypothalamus is a nuclear structure of the brain and in man is located above the roof of the mouth. The hypothalamus is made up of many sub-nuclei each of which appears to have a specific function. In general terms, the function of the hypothalamus is to provide for the regulation of internal conditions in the body. There are hypothalamic nuclei concerned with the regulation of body temperature, water balance, feeding behavior, sexual activities, and the like. The hypothalamus has the prime responsibility for maintaining constant internal conditions in the light of changing external conditions; a function subserved under the concept of homeostasis.

The hypothalamus being a critical portion of the brain has, as you might expect, widespread interconnections with other brain re-

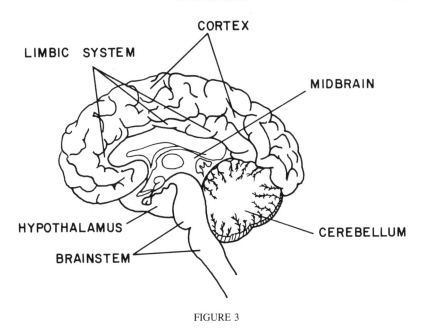

CORTEX

LIMBIC SYSTEM

MIDBRAIN

HYPOTHALAMUS

CEREBELLUM

BRAINSTEM

FIGURE 3

gions and is closely connected with the master endocrine gland, the pituitary. The hypothalamus and pituitary work in a very intimate and congenial relationship to provide for homeostatic control. The hypothalamus receives input from many portions of the body and brain regarding their state and has the primary role of maintaining constant internal conditions in the face of perturbations. The first means by which it accomplishes this is by direct neural control to other brain regions thereby adjusting behavior in the light of perturbing conditions. A second means of control is the ability of the hypothalamus to direct the pituitary gland to release endocrine hormones.

Mid-brain. The hypothalamus is a portion of the mid-brain. Another structure in the mid-brain is the reticular formation. This is a diffuse structure running up through the brain stem and ending in the mid-brain and consists of several components. One of the components receives sensory information from various sensory organs. This component of the reticular formation sends axons out to activate extensive areas of the neocortex. Electrical stimulation of this diffusely projecting system has been shown to awaken sleeping animals. Surgical destruction of this area produces continual sleep. This has led to the conceptualization of the reticular formation as being involved in arousal, waking and sleeping. Other components of reticular formation project in the opposite direction, that is, they influence principal cell activity in the spinal cord.

Subcortical area. Proceeding "upward," one encounters a vast number of subcortical structures. These are nuclear structures located, as the term implies, beneath the cortex. We will mention only the most obvious of these structures and those most relevant to our concerns. The thalamus is a large structure which is subdivided into smaller nuclei. Its primary function is the relaying of sensory information to the cortex. As the major sensory relay in the brain it contains nuclei for each of the senses. Some aspects of sensory processing occur at the level of the thalamus. Animals deprived of cortical sensory tissue are capable of responding only to gross aspects of the sensory world—such as intensity and frequency. The fine patterning of the sensory world is totally unavailable to them.

Limbic system. The other subcortical area of interest to us is not a single structure but rather a widespread but interconnected series of nuclei known as the limbic system. The limbic system is a somewhat mysterious portion of the brain in that despite concerted effort by many individuals its function still remains elusive. The results of experiments suggest that the limbic system is concerned with emotionality, with memory storage, and perhaps with learning. Some of the structures that comprise the limbic system are the amygdala, the hippocampus, and the septum.

Cerebral Cortex. The termination of our quick anatomical tour of the brain brings us to the cerebral cortex, also termed neocortex. The cerebral cortex, like many of the structures already considered is symetrically divided into a left and a right portion termed cerebral hemispheres. As has been mentioned earlier the cortex like other brain structures is composed of neurons and the axons that interconnect them and is highly fissured or convoluted.

The cortex is traditionally defined in terms of the four lobes that comprise it. These are the frontal, parietal, temporal, and occipital. Each of these lobes is associated with a primary sensory or motor function.

The *frontal lobes* contains neurons whose axons project down into the spinal cord to synapse on spinal motor neurons. Within the frontal motor area are represented all the muscles of the body. The neurons are not haphazardly scattered throughout the cortex, but rather exist in a distorted representation of the human body known as the motor homunculus. Stimulation delivered to this region of the cortex will produce movements or twitches in the appropriate musculature.

The *parietal lobe* of the cortex contains the somatic sensory receiving area. In this area are located neurons which receive inputs from the body senses of touch, pressure and temperature. Represented within the somatic sensory cortical area is a transformation of the receptor surface, in this case the surface of the body. As in the motor area, the sensory homunculus is distorted due to the fact that skin receptors are unequally represented across the surface of the skin. The lips and tongue as well as the hand of man have the highest density of sensory receptors and thus receive the greatest share of cortical space.

The *temporal lobe* contains the auditory areas. Represented within these areas is the receptor surface, in this case, the cochlea of the ear.

The *occipital lobe* contains the primary visual sensory receiving area of the cortex; here too, the receptor surface, the retina of the eye, is represented spatially on the surface of the visual cortex.

Within each of the four lobes of the human brain there exist large areas that are not devoted to sensory or motor events. These areas are termed *association areas*. Historically, the term association cortex referred to the belief that associations between stimuli or between stimulus and response were made in these regions of the brain. Currently, it is believed that the association cortex contains the neural machinery that enables the higher mental processing that distinguishes humans from our fellow creatures.

The cerebral cortex is only several millimeters thick, but contains within it several distinct layers. Some of these layers receive sensory information relayed by the thalamus from the sensory organs. Other layers contain the principle cells of the cortex that are sending their axons out of the cortex, either to subcortical structures or the principle cells in the spinal cord and thus to the musculature. Other regions contain local circuit neurons whose function is to modulate and integrate information within a limited area of cortex.

The association cortex apparently functions neither as sensory cortex, nor as a motor area; rather it seems to be involved with complex discriminations as well as those neural events that are associated with governing our behavior in accordance with external demands. A clue to its function comes from observing the relative amounts of association cortex across a wide variety of organisms. The common laboratory rat has only a miniscule amount of association cortex; the cat and dog have considerably more but nothing like the vast amount of association cortex found in the brains of the primate species, particularly the human brain. We assume that the brain functions underlying higher mental abilities, including language, are represented by association cortex to a large degree. However, our knowledge of the precise functions of association cortex is fragmentary and clearly much work needs to be done in order for us to gain a clear understanding of its precise functions.

To recapitulate, we have seen that the basic building block of the brain is the neuron, a cell little changed across species. Similarly we have seen that certain aspects of the organization of the brain have changed little across species, namely the spinal cord, and brain stem. The major difference across species is the tremendous expansion in association cortex which, coupled with a dramatic increase in the number of local circuit neurons and thus the kinds of processing that they are presumably engaged in, is primarily responsible for those attributes that distinguish the human species from our fellow inhabitants of this planet.

BRAIN DEVELOPMENT

A human fetus does not possess a miniature brain from the time of conception. Rather, the brain develops in quite distinct stages. Beginning as an undifferentiated piece of tissue, the brain is formed from a common class of precursor cells. At different times during the life of the embryo, the precursor cell population produces neurons destined to become specific tissues within the brain.

These features of brain development are important for several reasons. *Primary* among them being the fact that the fetus is extremely sensitive to drugs or toxic agents during this period of brain development. While generally protected from environment influences by the maternal placental barrier, the infant, however, can be affected by those chemicals and drugs capable of crossing the placental barrier. It is therefore critical that females, while pregnant, refrain from exposing themselves to drugs, medications, or toxic substances. The great danger is that we are unable to adequately identify all agents of potential danger to the developing brain of the fetus. In the inadvertent exposure to chemicals presumed to be safe but which are, in fact, damaging to the fetal brain lies the real danger. For these reasons, the prudent expectant mother should refrain from even such seemingly innocuous substances as prepared foods, which contain high quantities of artificial flavorings, artificial colorings, and preservatives generally of unknown effect on the developing brain of the child.

The *second aspect* of brain development that is important to consider is that the fetal brain is being built from the food provided to it by the mother. The human body is not capable of providing all of the necessary amino acids required for the building of proteins. Those materials that the body is capable of constructing (amino acids and fats, or lipids, that are essential to brain functioning), require the presence of adequate amounts of raw materials (molecules). These raw materials, or precursors, are obtained from the diet. A diet inadequate in the necessary precursors for lipids and amino acids may be reflected in a deficient fetal central nervous system. The situation may not be as critical as it first appears since the demands of the developing fetus are quite imperative and if the precursors are not supplied in the diet, the fetus may simply take them from the mother's own body. However, this must be considered an extreme reaction to dietary deficiency rather than the norm.

It therefore becomes quite important that mothers enjoy adequate nutrition during pregnancy and that young children continue to eat well-balanced meals until that period of time when the brain development slows down considerably. The human brain has completed most of its neuron cell production at birth but during the next four years increases in weight some 400%, most of this due to the expansion of the dendrites and axons of the neurons as well as to the elaboration of supporting cells of the brain. Therefore, during this period of time, and following until puberty, proper nutrition is quite important. In the following paragraphs, we shall consider some aspects of brain nutrition as they impact both on the fetus and on the developing child.

The Brain Dietary Requirements

We have seen that the developing brain depends on neuronal cell division and development over a lengthy time. Undernutrition in laboratory rats leads to a distortion of their patterns of connectivity. Behavioral measures of undernourished rats reflect this altered brain development. If not corrected, the changes are permanent. Nutritional rehabilitation, however, can undo many of the effects of early undernourishment. A similar picture emerges from studies done on undernourished children. They too are intellectually handicapped by a deficient diet during the formative stages of brain development. Thankfully, many of their deficiencies can also be reversed by later adequate nutrition. This is possible due to the remarkably adaptive properties of the brain, properties (termed "plasticity") that underlie learning and memory as well.

One of the brain neurotransmitters is *serotonin*. Serotonin has been linked to emotional behavior, sleep and reproductive behavior. It is synthesized from the amino acid tryptophan. One of the essential amino acids, tryptophan cannot be synthesized by humans and must be supplied in the foods we eat (bananas are loaded with tryptophan). If tryptophan is not supplied to a developing brain, serotonin synapses in the brain will be affected. Other transmitters require different substrates, but ultimately all of the precursors must be supplied by the foods eaten.

Another example of a dietary requirement for a neurotransmitter is acetylcholine, the transmitter at the nerve-muscle synapse as well as within the brain. Acetylcholine synthesis requires choline as one of its precursors. Choline must be obtained from the diet and is particularly abundant in egg yolk and certain vegetables such as soybeans. It has been discovered that some of the senile diseases of the aged are relieved by increasing the dietary intake of choline, through eating foods high in choline.

While it would be possible to devise "the brain diet," it is probably sufficient to recognize the critical role that nutrition plays in brain and thus intellectual habits for both mother and child. Clearly poor nutrition will influence a child's cognitive development.

INTEGRATIVE BRAIN FUNCTIONS

We have briefly examined the basic plan of the vertebrate brain and have spent some time considering the features and operations of the neuron—the basic building block of the brain. We have also examined some of the sensory, motor, and integrative processes in the brain. In this section we will consider some additional features of brain organization that we shall term integrative functions. By this we mean those attributes of the brain that are added upon the basic structure we have already mentioned and that show an interesting progression across species that parallels their behavioral capabilities.

Specialization

The maturing nervous system develops out of an undifferentiated neural tube. As the brain matures, neurons congregate into distinct regions and take on unique identifiable forms which are thought to be related to their function. The process of neuronal differentiation continues throughout gestation and forms the basis of the anatomical distinctions reviewed earlier. The emerging specialization of regions of the nervous system is much more finely tuned than can be appreciated from studying the gross structure of the brain. Within the layers of the cortex appear anatomically and, presumably, functionally distinct types of neurons. It is a dictum in biology that form and function go together.

Thus we note that the brain proceeds from a relatively undifferentiated mass of neural tissue into a quite specialized organ system. Contained within the mature brain are numerous subdivisions and subdivisions within subdivisions. It is one of the future tasks of the neurosciences to discern the functional distinctions between neuron types. We know that it is the patterns of neuronal activity among millions of neurons interacting in complex ways that make up our perception of the external world as well as our cognitive evaluation and response to these perceptions.

Lateralization

The brain is a symmetrical organ; just as you have two arms, you have two hemispheres which are mirror images of each other. At least this was the view of the organization of the brain until relatively recently. In the last decade it became apparent that the two hemispheres of the neocortex are neither anatomically symmetrical or functionally symmetrical. Actually, such asymmetries have been noted for approximately a hundred years, dating from the earliest observations of language impairment following damage to the left hemisphere and a relative lack of language impairment following damage to the right hemisphere. Excellent discussions of hemispheric laterality or specialization have appeared in a score of recent books, some of which are listed at the end of this chapter. Through a variety of diagnostic procedures (including CAT and PET scans) it is found that the functions of the dominant and nondominant hemispheres of the human brain and indeed of the brains of other primates are not identical. In excess of 90% of the human population can be considered right handed. For these individuals their dominant hemisphere is almost always the left. The remainder of the population, left handers and ambidextrous individuals, are found to have their dominant hemisphere in either the right or the left side of the brain, and in a very small number of cases appear to share dominance between the right and left side of the brain. While the assigning of dominance to one of the two hemispheres is not an easy task the general outlines of the distribution of functions between the two hemispheres is relatively clear.

The dominant hemisphere has been found to be that concerned with the understanding and production of language, computational and numerical abilities, and logical analytic and symbolic processes. The nondominant hemisphere appears to be specialized for perception of spatial and temporal relations, visual imagery, music (melodic) processing, and other nonverbal functions. It must be emphasized at the outset that these are not the exclusive functions of their respective hemispheres. Indeed, when one is speaking it does not follow that the nondominant hemisphere "turns off" and simply idles. Rather, one should view the two hemispheres and their respective specializations as systems that share many features in common but that are specialized for certain aspects of information processing. The two hemispheres are connected by a massive fiber bundle, the *corpus callosum*. This fiber system serves to interconnect the two hemispheres and presumably allows for the integration of the specialized processing capabilities of the right and left hemispheres.

The most dramatic studies that have been reported are those dealing with split-brained humans. Foremost among the neuroscientists working with these patients is the Nobelist Roger Sperry (1968). In a small number of humans suffering from epilepsy the corpus callosum was severed to control the spread of the disease, thus separating the two hemispheres. Through an extensive series of tests, it was shown that the above generalizations regarding hemispheric specializations could be seen in these patients, although in non-testing situations they appeared remarkably normal. Less dramatic (and less drastic) confirmation of these results have come from studies of intact human beings measuring the electrical activity from the surface of the scalp. Many of these studies have focused on some aspect of linguistic asymmetries. Other studies also employing EEG recording techniques and PET scans have demonstrated asymmetries in the brain electrical response that are associated with the performance of certain tasks, for example, listening to music or performing calculations.

These studies on hemispheric lateralization can be viewed as a further example of specialization in the brain. They have also opened up an interesting area of speculation regarding the modes of consciousness that are operative in the human brain.

GENETIC INFLUENCES

Readers may be aware of the work of the Nobel Laureates David Hubel and Torsten Wiesel (1963) describing the high degree of stimulus specificity shown by single neurons in the visual area of the cortex. Briefly, the output from the retina projects to the visual portion (lateral geniculate) of the thalamus (the major sensory relay center of the brain) and thus to the visual area of the cortex (the striate cortex). Neurons in the striate cortex respond to quite specific stimuli in the visual world-lines, edges, bias, moving wedges, etc., depending upon where in the striate cortex one is.

In a landmark experiment, Hubel and Wiesel demonstrated that these neurons did not acquire this specificity as a result of interacting with a visual world. Their experiment involved recording from kittens whose eyes were first opened to view the moving bars, etc., of the laboratory. Clearly these animals did not have an opportunity to benefit from the visual world. Yet, their neurons responded in the same way to the patterned stimuli as did those of adult cats. The role of heredity in establishing this high degree of sensory decoding has thus been established. This is not to say that the environment plays no role in the development of the brain's capacity to process visual information—far from it. There exists an extensive literature that has examined just this interaction between heredity and environment. While the most detailed information exists for the visual system, it appears that the other sensory modalities operate along similar lines.

For our purposes there are two points of interest in the above. First, a good deal of "processing" occurs in the input or sensory system, and second, much of the brain's response to visual information has been initially determined by our genes and subsequently modified by our environment.

For example, psycholinguists have established that certain speech sounds are perceived categorically. That is, instead of perceiving a continuum of sounds, as in musical pitch, the listener categorizes these sounds, into two categories which differ in voice onset. Since categorical perception of human speech sounds is also seen in nonverbal animals, it probably represents sensory processing in the brain, as opposed to learning.

At this juncture, it is an open question as to what other (if any) aspects of language are defined by the peculiarities of the brain. We, here, are not referring to the obvious restrictions such as the pitch of voice, the rapidity of speech, or its loudness. These are obvious constraints imposed by the physiology of our brain and sensory transducers. Rather we wonder about the syntax, semantics and content of language as determined by brain processes.

The second point, that there exists a sizable genetic component in sensory processing, is also relevant to human behavior. Obviously genetics plays an essential role in that the basic structure and function of our body and brain are genetically specified. Just as with categorical perception in language, our brain systems (particularly sensory systems) are specified to respond to certain aspects of the world as in the Hubel and Wiesel experiments. Furthermore it is the interaction of the brain with its environment that ultimately determines brain function and behavior.

SUMMARY

We have seen in this chapter that the organ of behavior, the human brain, is composed of billions of complicated neurons. Each neuron acts like a tiny computer, integrating the information sent to it and producing its own response to that input. That response, its action potential, is in turn sent to thousands of other neurons in a complicated web of information processing.

Neuroscientists are far from understanding the details of complicated information processing but, as will be considered in the chapter on Higher Brain Functions, are beginning to make inroads into this fascinating realm of brain function. What they do know a great deal about is the operation of the single neuron, the nature of synaptic interactions and the chemistry of neurotransmission. The future of the neurosciences is quite clear. Topics once considered the exclusive province of the psychologist, such as learning, memory, perception and motivation, will increasingly come under the scrutiny of the neuroscientist. The lessons for the educator in this are equally clear. As the brain processes that underlie things critical to education are gradually understood, the educator will be in an enviable position to profit from these discoveries to the great benefit of the student.

REFERENCES CITED

Hubel, D. H. and Wiesel, T. N. Receptive fields of cells in striate cortex of very young, visually inexperienced kittens. *Journal of Neurophysiology*, 1963, *26*, 994-1002.
Sperry, R. W. Hemisphere deconnections and unity in conscious awareness. *American Psychologist*, 1968, *23*, 723-733.

SUGGESTIONS FOR FURTHER READING

Teyler, T.J. *A Primer of Psychobiology, 2nd Edition,* Freeman: San Francisco, 1983.
Thompson, R.F. *Introduction to Physiological Psychology,* Harper & Row: New York, 1975.
The Brain, A Scientific American Book, Freeman: San Francisco, 1979.
Wittrock, M. D. (Editor). *The Human Brain,* Prentice-Hall: New York, 1977.
Springer, S.P. and Deutsch, G. *Left Brain, Right Brain,* Freeman: San Francisco, 1981.

Higher Brain Function

N. L. Chiaia, MA
T. J. Teyler, PhD

ABSTRACT. In this chapter we examine higher mental function in the brain, and the developmental processes which influence them. Environmental factors operate in three major areas: 1) information input via the sensory and perceptual systems, 2) information organization, and 3) behavioral output. Developmental and environmental factors which affect brain information in each of these areas is reviewed with the intent of acquainting the reader with the major principles of brain-behavior organization. In the final section we discuss the physiological alterations in brain function as it relates to major clinical syndromes.

INTRODUCTION

As educators, the readers of this journal are faced daily with the functioning, and sometimes dysfunctioning, person interacting with the environment in a learning situation. Your commitment as educators is to the transmission of information in a fashion so organized that the information might be used by the recipient in the future to optimize interactions with the environment. It is of importance to the educator to have some global understanding of the mental machinery responsible for the ability to acquire and integrate and use information. All of this might be subsumed under the general rubric of "learning."

The question of "how learning works" is fundamental among the behavioral and social sciences and more recently has found itself the object, at a more molecular level, of investigations in the field of basic neuroscience. From this standpoint the concerns of the educator overlap with those of the neuroscientist. Both are concerned, albeit at different levels, with the mechanisms by which

N. L. Chiaia and T. J. Teyler are affiliated with the Neurobiology Program, Northeastern Ohio Universities College of Medicine, Rootstown, OH 44272.

we acquire, process and transmit information gathered through interaction with our environment. Though the basic neurosciences are still quite far from a complete understanding of the basic mechanisms underlying learning and memory, some significant strides have been made in our thinking. The explosion of information in the neurosciences in recent years is astounding and challenges the ability of even the most widely read professional to keep pace with new developments. It is the purpose of this chapter to discuss some of the recent developments in the neurosciences relevant to the field of education, namely, advances in our understanding of higher brain function.

Most of the data from which the following discussion has been drawn comes from research completed in several prominent animal laboratories around the country. While caution must be exercised in applying the principles garnered from investigations in animals directly to humans, it is our contention that the general principles found to govern learning in animals will serve to direct investigations of these phenomenon in humans.

This chapter is divided into three major sections. In the first section we will deal principally with the neural processes and environmental factors which effect information input. The input of information into the neural machinery is an important area of research. The sensory and perceptual channels through which information enters the brain system can be influenced by a number of factors. The type and amount of incoming information can in turn exert a profound effect on neuronal architecture. In addition, we will examine the role of environmental factors and environmental enrichment in the development of perceptual and learning abilities.

In the second section we will deal with some aspects of information storage and processing and some current research which support them. We will discuss what is presently known about the neural mechanisms of information coding and storage and the organization and flow of information through the brain. Finally we will review how what is currently known about the pathways of information input and distribution within the brain and how these data support some of the current models of information processing developed by cognitive psychologists.

In the final section, we will deal with the damaged or dysfunctional brain and the neurobiological manifestations of dysfunction in some prevalent childhood disorders.

INFORMATION INPUT AND REGISTRATION
IN THE BRAIN

Development and Sensory Coding

The major path of input of information from the environment to our brain is via sensory systems. Humans possess several classes of specialized sense organs which respond to specific types of physical energy in the environment. These sense organs, or sensory receptors, are responsible for receiving certain types of physical stimuli (energy) and transforming (tranducing) this energy into electrochemical impulses for subsequent processing in the brain. The visual receptors, for example, are sensitive to electromagnetic radiation in the form of light energy. Energy is received in the retina of the eye and transformed into electrical impulses which are then transmitted through the visual sensory channel, eventually arriving at the occipital area of the cerebral cortex. The end result is the experience of sight. In other words a physical stimulus from the environment is transformed into a pattern of neural activity in specific parts of the nervous system. This pattern of neural activity is termed the *"afferent code."* Sensory neurobiology is a branch of the neurosciences devoted to investigating the afferent codes for stimuli in the sensory systems.

Investigators in the field of sensory neurobiology have made some surprising discoveries about the afferent codes for different types of stimuli, particularly in the visual system. They have observed that different classes of neurons in the visual cortex of cats and monkeys are capable of extracting different types of information from an image in the visual world. One class of neurons is capable of responding to the presence or absence of a simple spot of light. A second, more complex class of cells, responds to lines or bars of light oriented in a particular direction (vertical, horizontal), a third class of cells responds only to bars of light moving in a specific direction across the visual field. These latter two types of afferent codes are termed "orientation selectivity" and "directional selectivity." These different types of information are extracted by different classes of neurons in the visual cortex. Other types of information relating to color and intensity of light are extracted by neurons at the level of the thalamic relay neurons as well as by cortical neurons. It is the sum total of all of this information processing regarding color, orientation, direction and movement that results in a visual experience or visual sensation. The situation has been found to be much the same in other sensory systems. Separate classes of neurons in the auditory system have been found to code information regarding the pitch, loudness and location of sound. Similarly, separate neurons in the somatosensory system are responsible for extracting information about the position and intensity of tactile stimuli and temperature.

In the previous chapter we noted that the ability of specific classes of neural elements to respond to different aspects of stimuli could be observed even in perceptually naive animals. Such an observation shows that there is a strong genetic component to this capacity. Research in sensory neurobiology in the past decade has shown, however, that early environmental interaction may exert equally powerful influences over the response properties of neurons in the sensory systems. Research done at Cambridge University by Colin Blakemore (1970) in kittens has suggested that the type of visual environment to which an animal is exposed plays a dramatic role in both neural and behavioral responses. In these experiments, kittens were reared in restricted visual environments containing only lines and stripes of either vertical or horizontal orientation. When examined behaviorally in adulthood these animals exhibited profound deficits in their ability to maneuver in an environment which contained objects whose plane of orientation was orthogonal to that of the environment in which the animal was reared. Cats reared in a "vertical" environment were consistently observed bumping into horizontal object (table tops) and animals reared in a "horizontal" environment experienced similar difficulties with vertically oriented objects (table legs). The animals behaved as if they "just did not see" some of the objects in front of them.

These observations prompted experimenters to examine the response properties of neurons in the visual cortex of these animals. What they found was dramatic. Neurons in the visual cortex of these animals demonstrated a marked preference for responding to objects of the same orientation of the environment in which they were reared. They had few neural elements capable of responding to visual stimuli of the opposite orientation. In effect, restricted visual experience during development had significantly altered the type of information extracted from the environment by neural elements in the visual system.

Further experiments were performed with monkeys raised from birth with translucent occluders placed over the eyes. These occluders allowed diffuse light to register on the retina but prevented any pattern or form vision. Animals raised in this fashion displayed profound deficits in form, pattern and depth perception as adults. Similar deficits have been observed in human infants with cataract occlusion of the retina. If corrective surgery in these infants is not performed very early in development, perceptual difficulties will persist throughout adulthood. It appears that there can be no adequate substitute for early environmental interaction in shaping sensory systems.

Learning, Plasticity and Constancy in Perception

We have seen that environmental interaction plays a critical role in the developing organism in shaping the type of information extracted from the environment by the brain. The organization of sensory information into coherent perceptions is also subject to the effects of environmental interactions. Much of what we perceive daily has been programmed by experience with the environment. In addition, we have already seen that the structure of our brain imposes certain constraints on the type of information to which we are capable of responding. How we organize sensations into complex perceptions is a process that is not well understood. The nature versus nurture controversy rages quite violently in this area of perceptual psychology. There is, however, good evidence to support the important role of "learning" in the organization of perceptions.

The world as we perceive it is a relatively stable commodity, although the actual physical stimuli which impinge upon our sensory receptors are constantly changing. As we move about in space our perceptions of the world and objects around us remain constant. For example, the retinal image of an object increases in size as we approach it, yet we do not perceive the object as actually getting larger. Similarly the color of an object does not appear to change if the object is viewed under differing illuminations, yet we know that the physical properties of the retinal image are not the same under different lighting conditions. What then accounts for our ability to organize different physical stimuli into relatively "constant" perceptions?

Current research in the field of perceptual constancies proposes that as we develop, our interactions with our environment allow us to adopt a set of perceptual strategies which direct the way in which we organize incoming sensory information. In the case of size and color constancy stated above, it has been shown that the important factor is not quality or intensity or any single stimulus in an image, but rather the "relationship" of each element of the stimulus array to all of the other elements. Thus if the size increase in the retinal image of an object which we are approaching is not significantly different from the increase in the retinal image for other objects in the visual scene then the perceptual decision which will result is that "we are moving in space with respect to this particular object." If, on the other hand, only the object of interest appears to change in size and surrounding objects remain the same we will most probably decide that the object of interest is now moving with respect to us. The mechanisms by which we adopt these "relational" perceptual strategies are not thoroughly understood, but their existence is undeniable.

A somewhat more complex example of the use of perceptual strategies is our ability to perceive "depth" in a photograph or drawing which contains only two dimensions. Clearly the stimuli present in an actual visual image differ from those contained in a photograph of the same scene, yet we perceive a three dimensional image in both cases. We are only beginning to understand the perceptual and relational rules which allow us to accomplish this.

We now turn our attention to the notion of plasticity in perceptual experience. We have seen that both the structure of our brain and developmentally learned "strategies" interact to allow the human to achieve some measure of constancy in the perception. Drastic alterations in sensory input produced by artificial means can present problems for our sensory and perceptual apparatus. Our sensory systems possess a remarkable ability to adapt to the reorganization of incoming stimuli. A series of ingenious experiments done at the University of Austria by Ivo Kohler demonstrates this remarkable ability. In these experiments human subjects were fitted with special prismatic goggles which inverted the visual image such that the entire visual world appeared upside-down. Significant orientation problems were experienced by subjects wearing these goggles in their attempts to navigate through their environment. After a period of several weeks of wearing the prism goggles, however, most of the subjects found that they were able to function quite well and, in fact, began to report that the world no longer felt as if it were upside-down. The perceptual machinery in these individuals appeared to be capable of reorganizing visual and kinesthetic information so that normal sensorimotor integration was possible. In many of these cases, it was reported that removal of the goggles after several weeks resulted again in a period of disorientation before which the world again looked "normal." The ability of the perceptual system to adapt to these drastically altered sensory images seemed particularly dependent upon active interaction with the environment. Subjects who were prevented from actively exploring their environment through voluntary movements were unable to adapt to the effect of the prisms and could never make the "world look right."

So far we have discussed a number of factors which can affect the registration, organization and interpretation of sensory input into the brain. Though these processes are complex and their neural correlates are far from being fully understood they provide us with a framework in which to view general patterns of normal perceptual functioning. The reader should now more fully appreciate that our day-to-day perceptions are by no means a simple or even faithful reproduction of the physical stimuli which bombard us. Rather they are the result of a complex filtering system whose operations are not fixed rigidly at birth but subject to alteration through physical maturation and interaction with the environment. The consequences of disruption of the normal operation of this filtering system and the extent to which such disruptions contribute to a variety of organic brain syndromes is largely unknown. It is hoped that as the gap between the basic sciences and the clinical sciences is bridged more progress will be made in these areas.

THE EFFECTS OF ENVIRONMENTAL ENRICHMENT ON BRAIN STRUCTURE AND LEARNING

We have cited examples of the complex interaction of environmental experience and perceptual processing in modulating the input of information to the central nervous system. If it is true that environmental interaction can modulate the development and function of central neural processes, which in turn can modulate behavior, then one might presume that the greater the amount of positive environmental interactions available to an organism during development the more optimal should be its development. Early research in the area of environmental enrichment and its effects on brain function and behavior attempted to address two very basic questions: 1. Does exposure to an "enriched" versus an "impoverished" environment early in development result in any measurable enhancement in brain development? 2. If so what is the nature and developmental time course of the effect?

The standard environmental enrichment experiment utilized three experimental groups. One group was exposed to an optimized or "enriched" environment, while a second group was exposed to an "impoverished" environment and finally a third group was exposed to a standard laboratory environment and served as a reference or "control" group. During the past decade many experiments have been done in rodents utilizing this paradigm and it would be impossible to review all the pertinent findings in the confines of this chapter. In general, the results of these studies found that exposure to an enriched environment early in the development produced marked effects in three areas: (a) brain morphology, (b) brain biochemistry, and (c) learning ability.

The brains of the enriched animals were found to exhibit significantly increased weight in certain brain areas, particularly sensory areas. At the microscopic level, enriched animals possessed slightly larger cells, especially in the sensory areas, as well as an increase in the number and complexity of the dendritic outgrowth from these cells. With respect to brain biochemistry, enriched animals exhibited higher levels of the neurotransmitter acetylcholine as well as enhanced manufacturing of brain proteins. Behaviorally these animals were found to be superior to both their impoverished and control littermates on several laboratory learning tasks including; maze learning, discrimination and reversal learning, and both passive and active avoidance. The magnitude of these effects was found to be directly correlated with the length of exposure of the animal to the enriched environment as well as the age of the animal at the time of exposure. Longer exposures of several months produced the best effect and the effects were most pronounced in pre-weaning animals. Due to both practical and ethical constraints such experiments cannot be performed in humans and it is therefore difficult to know what extent these results apply to humans, as well as what factors would constitute an "enriched" human environment. Nevertheless, such studies were, in part, responsible for the creation of governmental programs like Head Start, which were designed to optimize the early learning environment of children.

LEARNING, MEMORY AND HIGHER MENTAL FUNCTION

Earlier we dealt with the mechanism and channels for the input of information into the CNS from the environment. Getting information into the brain, however, is only the first step. The information which has been entered must be processed further and stored in some fashion for future use. The time course of the storage may be short term, in anticipation of immediate use, or it may be relatively permanent. The mental processes which now become operative are quite varied and complex. We shall deal here with only a small subset of them. We will restrict our discussion to those mechanisms involved in the storage and retrieval of information as well as the mechanism of attention and arousal by which the organism is readied for learning. Finally, we will deal with the more complex issues of what is known about the physiological correlates of cognitive processes.

Learning and Memory: Animal Models

The processes by which we learn and remember have been the subject of investigation in the field of physiological psychology for several decades. During this time there has been little agreement as to what approach is most appropriate with respect to gaining some insight into those processes most important to humans. Some researchers in the field of learning contend that humans represent the pinnacle of evolutionary development by virtue of their ability to fashion and use tools and their development of a unique communication system in the form of language. Language plays an important role in the processing, organization and retrieval of information in humans. These researchers propose that human memorial and learning processes are unique and cannot be adequately modeled by species that do not possess the same cognitive and linguistic capacities. It is our contention, and that of many other neurobiologists, that the physiological laws which govern learning and the neuronal substrates which underlie them are independent of the cognitive capacities of language. This statement should not be interpreted as a disregard for the role of linguistic and cognitive factors in human memory, but rather an attempt to adopt a simplified approach to the study of information acquisition and storage.

Learning and memory at the neuronal level may operate through similar mechanisms in both animals and man. Though there is some disagreement, most psychologists would agree that the fundamental factors which control the acquisition of behavioral responses are quite similar in both humans and animals. There is little reason to believe that the neuronal mechanisms which underlie these processes are different.

Fruitful investigations of the molecular mechanisms of learning and memory require the use of intrusive techniques which cannot be used in humans, necessitating the need for animal models. These models typically examine simple forms of learning such as "habituation," "sensitization" and "classical conditioning" in simple animals.

Habituation refers to a decrease in the strength of the behavioral response to a given stimulus as a function of repeated presentation of that stimulus. It is considered by many to be the most elemental form of learning. The responses of neurons to sensory stimulation from the environment and to electrical stimulation in the laboratory have been shown to exhibit habituation. The cellular mechanisms responsible for neural habituation are quite complex and beyond the scope of this chapter, but it is hoped that the discovery of the neural processes responsible for habituation will shed further light on the molecular mechanisms of learning.

Classical conditioning is another behavioral paradigm that has proved extremely useful for the study of learning at the molecular level. In this paradigm two stimuli are repeatedly presented in close temporal contiguity to an organism. One of the stimuli normally possess the ability to elicit a reflexive response upon presentation. The other stimulus elicits no response. Through the repeated, temporally-contiguous pairing of the stimuli, the neutral stimulus gradually acquires the ability to elicit the reflexive response. Richard Thompson (1976), at Stanford University, is examining the electrical activity of the rabbit brain during the acquisition of a classically conditioned response. Dramatic changes in brain activity have been observed during conditioning and have been shown to correlate precisely with the change in behavior.

Models of Memory: The Amnesia Paradigm

Loss of memory for events just prior to physical or psychological trauma is a well documented human phenomenon. "Amnesia" is reported for events ranging from minutes to hours prior to the traumatizing incident. Clinically, profound memory deficits have been observed in neurological patients who have sustained damage to the temporal lobe of the brain, particularly in the limbic system (see previous chapter). Temporal lobe resection is a surgical procedure which is sometimes performed in severe cases of epilepsy in an attempt to reduce the severity and frequency of epileptic seizures. The severity of the side effects of this surgery on epileptic patients precludes its widespread use. Such patients exhibit a particular inability to retain recently learned information, but have no difficulty remembering events which occurred years earlier. One classic patient (H.M.) has been observed to read the same magazines day after day without ever remembering the contents of his reading.

In order to study the processes responsible for memory loss, psychobiologists have attempted to construct an animal model of amnesia. Temporal lobe damage has been induced in laboratory animals. These animals demonstrate severe deficits in their ability to acquire simple behavioral responses. This impairment is observed across a wide variety of learning tasks including both classical and instrumental learning, as well as avoidance tasks. Brain lesion models are not the only models which have been developed for the study of memory. A recent model called the Experimental Amnesia Paradigm (Figure I) has proved to be of great value. The experimental amnesia paradigm involves producing a loss of memory for a previously learned behavior through the controlled application of a traumatizing treatment or agent. A variety of amnestic agents have been found to be effective in producing amnesia. They fall into three categories: 1) electrical-consisting of pulses of electric shock to the brain, 2) chemical-consisting of injection of a variety of pharmacological agents, and 3) metabolic-consisting of alterations in metabolism induced through hypothermia. The brain mechanism through which amnestic treatments operate has been the source of controversy.

Memory Stages and the Trace Theory of Memory

Classically, the process of formulating a memory has been thought to occur in three distinct stages (Figure 2). Sensory information comes into the organism's nervous system and its presence is recorded in the "sensory register." From here the information is transferred to a second "short term" storage phase in anticipation of immediate use or further elaboration and processing. Finally, information that is to be earmarked for retrieval at some future

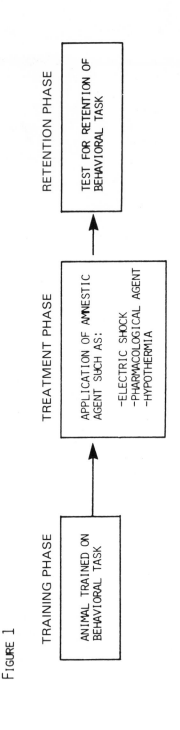

FIGURE 1

EXPERIMENTAL AMNESIA PARADIGM

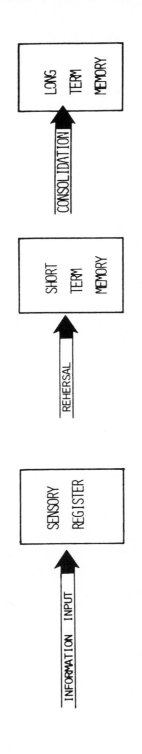

FIGURE 2

SENSORY REGISTER

INFORMATION INPUT

SHORT TERM MEMORY

REHERSAL

LONG TERM MEMORY

CONSOLIDATION

STAGE MODEL OF MEMORY

time is transferred from the short term store to a third "long term" phase. It is the transfer of information from the "short term" store to the "long term" store that has occupied the attentions of most memory researchers.

The transfer of information from the short term to the long term store in the brain is a process known as "consolidation." The various amnestic treatments described earlier were thought to produce their effects by interfering with memory consolidation. These agents were typically applied to laboratory animals immediately following a training experience and were thought to produce an electrical or biochemical disruption which prevented the further processing of information, resulting in amnesia.

Consolidation or storage failure has recently become the subject of heated controversy in the field of memory. Recent evidence from animal learning laboratories suggest that amnesia may in fact result from an inability to retrieve information from long term storage. A number of investigators have observed that the amnesia caused by post-training application of a standard amnestic agent can be ameliorated by exposing the animal to some salient feature of the environment in which the learning occurred. This phenomenon is known as the "reminder" effect. The memory for the event apparently still exists in these animals but is not accessible to voluntary retrieval until the proper cues are provided. Memory loss in such instances appears to result from "retrieval failure" rather than "storage failure."

Proponents of this hypothesis classify memories into two categories, "active" or "inactive." Active memories are those which have achieved storage in the proper fashion and are amenable to immediate retrieval. Inactive memories are stored events which do not possess retrieval cues and thus are presently non-retrievable. It is possible for an inactive memory to become active when the appropriate retrieval cues are supplied. The critical parameters of effective retrieval cues are not fully understood.

The physiological state of an animal at the time of learning has recently been shown to have dramatic effects on retention. Animals trained to perform certain behavioral responses while in a particular physiological state or under the influence of certain drugs perform poorly or as if they were naive when tested for memory while in a different physiological state. In experiments conducted by Donald Overton (1964) at McGill University, rats were trained to turn toward the right arm of a T-shaped maze while under the influence of the barbiturate Sodium Pentothal. When the animals were later tested for the retention of this response in a non-drugged state they exhibited little evidence of memory for the task. If, however, the animals were tested for retention under the influence of the drug, they showed significant amounts of retention. The pharmacological state of these animals seemed to serve as a cuing mechanism for retrieval of the memory. This phenomenon is termed "state dependent learning." State dependent learning is probably an extreme example of the effectiveness of both internal and external cues to the indexing of memory.

Much research is currently being conducted on the role of environmental and "contextual cues" in information retrieval. A better understanding of how the brain tags information for later indexing the retrieval is of obvious significance to the field of education. For example it seems entirely possible that the critical factors which govern the efficient indexing of memories may exhibit some variability from situation to situation and from person to person. In our teaching experience we have seen that some students rely on text materials more heavily than lectures and other students rely more heavily on lectures than text materials. Aside from personal preferences, different cues and indexing strategies may be operative. Effective teaching requires the educator to become aware of possible differences in indexing strategies among pupils. This could be especially important in the area of special education and the teaching of learning impaired students. In addition the influences of chronic medication to brain injured students may affect the way in which information is tagged for later retrieval. These effects may require very careful scrutiny as they may be quite subtle.

Mechanisms of Memory Storage

We have discussed some of the processes which govern information processing and transfer during learning and memory but little has been said about the physical substrates of learning. Learning can be defined in its broadest sense as "a relatively permanent change in behavior as a function of experience." The behavioral change which occurs during learning must be mediated by a concomitant change in the brain. The question of "what changes in the brain during learning" is central to the field of neurobiology. Three major candidates for the neural substrate of learning which have been examined in recent years are: 1. biochemical factors, 2. electrophysiological factors, and 3. anatomical factors.

Support for the importance of biochemical factors in the formation of memory came from early work in invertebrate species. Experiments with flatworms showed that if biochemical extracts from a group of worms trained to perform a certain behavior were fed to naive worms, the naive worms were able to learn the task more quickly. Some factor present on the extract of trained worms appeared to enhance learning in naive worms. We have previously noted that environmental enrichment during development result in an enhanced capacity to learn as well as an increase in certain cellular chemicals (RNA and DNA) involved in the production of brain proteins. Proteins are large molecules that serve as structural and functional elements in the cells of many organs.

It is possible that the formation of proteins and their metabolic activity may play some role in the coding of memory in the brain. Experiments in several laboratories have shown that if drugs which impair protein manufacture in the brain are administered to an animal after the learning of a behavioral response, the memory for the response is diminished. More recently, increases in a certain type of brain protein have been observed in goldfish after learning. How the increases in these proteins are related to the learning or to the performance of the task is not yet clear.

The brain operates on biologically generated electrical impulses. It would be surprising if changes in these impulses did not accompany learning. The types of electrical activity present in the brain and the methods for their measurement are numerous. We will restrict ourselves to a brief description of the major types.

The most global measure of electrical activity in the brain is the Electroencephalogram (EEG) (Figure 3). This consists of a complex series of electrical waves recordable from the outer surface of the scalp in both human and animals. It is a complex electrical integration of activity from many areas of the brain at once. Changes in the patterns of EEG activity have been observed during learning by several laboratories. Unfortunately, the complexity of the EEG waves and the fact that they represent integrations of neural activity from many brain areas, make detection and localization of the source of the alteration in brain electrical activity difficult. For this reason many researchers have begun to look at the more restricted patterns of brain activity present in single neurons and small groups of neurons. Recording this type of brain activity requires

FIGURE 3

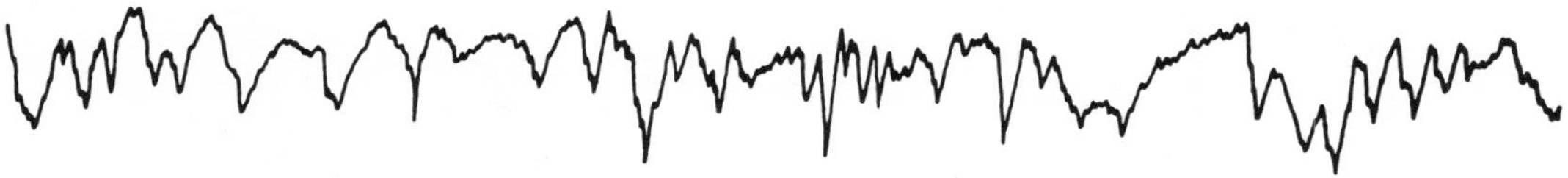

CORTICAL EEG

invasive techniques and can only be done in animals. Stanford's
Richard F. Thompson (1970) has reported some interesting
changes in both small group and single unit neural activity that, as
we have mentioned, is correlated with the acquisition of a classically conditioned blinking response in rabbits. Novel patterns of
neural activity appear as the response is learned and remain perma-
nently. These patterns do not appear in animals that are not
trained. It is interesting to note that the greatest changes have been
found in the Limbic System, an area we have already noted to be
implicated clinically in memory, and the cerebellum, a structure
heretofore thought to be involved exclusively with movement
coordination.

The search for the anatomical substrates of learning and memory is probably one of the oldest areas of research in neurobiology.
Early investigators attempted to define the locus of learning in the
brain by destroying various areas with lesions and observing the
effects of this destruction. Learning and memory were found to
survive surprising amounts of damage to large amounts of brain
tissue. To date, only two areas have been implicated in learning
deficit: the limbic system, as already mentioned, and certain areas
of the cerebral cortex. However, since learning clearly occurs in
organisms which do not possess these brain structures their importance to learning is not absolute and may be limited to the more
complex forms of learning. A more productive approach to the anatomical substrates of memory has been conducted at the level of
single neurons. Detectable changes in neuronal shape and connectivity have been reported in brains of trained animals. These
changes are subtle and their significance is not clear at present.

Arousal and Attention: Focusing the Neural Network

It should be obvious by now that all physical stimuli which impinge upon the brain do not result in behavioral output. Some
stimuli are excluded because the organism does not possess the
proper sensory receptors to detect them. Other stimulus information may be lost because existing receptor mechanisms are not adjusted or oriented to receive them.

In order to fully process stimuli, the neural network must be focused on the incoming stimulus. This directing of the processing
system is known as "attention." Attention is manifest behaviorally
by orienting the sensory receptors toward the source of the physi-

cal stimulus. This behavioral manifestation represents a class of behaviors known as orienting responses. Turning ones eyes toward a moving object in the distance, or a dog pricking its ears up at a novel sound are examples of common orienting responses. Orienting responses are elicited by stimuli of all sensory modalities.

Early investigations of orienting responses demonstrated that these responses are accompanied by marked changes in the EEG record through small electrodes placed on the scalp of an individual. The EEG of an awake but inattentive individual is characterized by a series of fairly regular "synchronized" patterns of neural activity called "alpha" waves. When a novel stimulus is presented to the individual, alpha waves are blocked and replaced by an "asynchronous" pattern of small amplitude fast activity called beta waves. This desynchronization of the cortical EEG is often used by behavioral investigators as an index of attention and has been found to correlate well with arousal in other physiological systems, such as heart rate and respiration. Stimuli of all sensory modalities are capable of producing desynchronization of the cortical EEG. Stimuli that are particularly important to given species do so more easily and persistently. In humans the primates visual stimuli are known to produce marked desynchronization, while olfactory stimuli seem to be more effective in mammals such as rodents.

The cortical EEG is not the only measure of electrical activity in the brain which exhibits changes correlated with attention. Changes have been observed in the activity of structures in the brain stem as well. The ability of an organism to attend to any stimulus is related to the state of wakefulness or arousal in the organism at the time the stimulus is encountered. Lesion experiments have shown that damage to certain areas of the brain stem result in an organism which is in a constant state of sleep. Electrical stimulation of the same structure produces a state of alert arousal. Changes have also been observed in the electrical activity of structures in the limbic system (see previous chapter) during the learning of complex behavioral tasks that requires the organism to pay close attention to specific environmental cues. When learning proceeds in these tasks it is accompanied by the appearance of a characteristic type of electrical activity called theta waves in the brain electrical records. There is some speculation that the appearance of theta waves signals that the given stimuli have acquired some saliency or meaning for the organism.

In contrast to the spontaneous brain activity recorded in the

EEG, electrical response may be recorded from the brain following the presentation of specific stimuli to the sensory receptors. These responses are termed *evoked potentials*. Records of three types of evoked potentials are shown in Figure 4. Alterations in evoked responses, particularly in their size have been shown to be correlated with attention. Clinical disorders which engender attentional deficits such as minimal brain dysfunction, autism, hyperkinesis, and mental retardation have been shown to exhibit abnormalities in evoked potentials.

Another example of evoked brain activity found to be correlated with attentional processes is a class of potentials known as *"expectancy waves."* A special paradigm is used to evoke these waves in humans. A subject is told that two stimuli will be presented in succession. The first stimulus is a warning stimulus (a flash of light, for example) and is used only to signal the impending occurrence of the second stimulus, the imperative stimulus. The subject is instructed to respond only to the imperative stimulus, but to use the warning stimulus in preparation to respond. The EEG of the subject is recorded in the interim between the warning stimulus and the imperative stimulus. Characteristic shifts in the baseline patterns of the EEG can be observed. It is thought that these shifts are related to the expectancy state created in the subject by the warning stimulus. The shifts are thus termed *"expectancy waves."* EEG desynchronization, cortical evoked potentials and expectancy waves are all areas of recent active research. It is hoped that finer analysis of these patterns of activity will provide a better understanding of the neural basis of attention and perhaps a useful diagnostic tool for the recognition of brain disorders.

Cognitive Constructs: Avenues of Processing

We have dealt with how information gets into the brain and the processes which select information for further analysis, i.e., the processes of sensation and attention. The complex psychological processing that determines the nature of thought and eventually knowledge is not well understood. Theories of the neural mechanisms of cognition are scarce. However, neurobiologists are beginning to decipher what are the most appropriate questions to pose and how best to go about answering them. Much of the significant work in recent years has been done in the cerebral cortex of the brain. The cerebral cortex has long been thought to be responsible

FIGURE 4

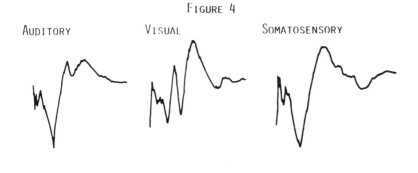

AUDITORY VISUAL SOMATOSENSORY

COMMON SENSORY EVOKED POTENTIALS

for higher cognitive functions. It is by far one of the most complex structures in the brain and the one about which the least is known. Neurobiologists in the past decade have been concerned with describing the anatomical organization of the cerebral cortex. A more thorough understanding of cortical organization may be the first step in deciphering the complex cognitive function for which it appears to be responsible. Insights are beginning to be gained into the way in which neural information is distributed within the cerebral cortex. We will precede our discussion of information distribution in the cortex with a brief look at cortical anatomy.

The cerebral cortical mantle consists of a thick blanket of neural tissue composed of six distinct layers of neurons, which covers the rest of the brain. The cortical mantle is composed of two symmetrical hemispheres each of which can be divided into four major areas or lobes. The anterior part of each hemisphere is the frontal lobe, the middle portion is the parietal lobe, the lateral portion is the temporal lobe and the posterior portion is the occipital lobe. The position of these lobes within the cerebral hemisphere can be seen in Figure 5. The three general types of cortical tissue, sensory, motor, and associational cortex, are housed within these lobes. Sensory cortex is responsible for receiving information from the sensory organs via the sensory relay areas of the thalamus (see previous chapter). The position of the primary sensory cortices for vision, audition, and somesthesis can be seen in Figure 6. The motor cortex (Figure 6 cross-hatched) is responsible for initiating mo-

FIGURE 5

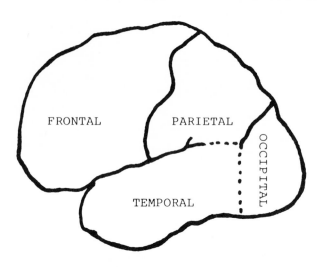

MAJOR LOBES OF THE CEREBRAL HEMISPHERES

tor commands to the body musculature for the production of voluntary movements. Association cortices are those areas which are not sensory or motor. It is thought that they serve as centers for higher cognitive processing and receive input from the sensory and motor cortices.

All cortical areas, regardless of their function, possess six distinct cellular layers. Within each layer reside specific classes of neurons. It is thought that the cellular composition of a given layer may be related to the way information is transmitted to and from that layer. Layers three and four of the cortex, for example, are primarily input layers which receive information from other parts of the cortex and from the sensory systems. Layers five and six, on the other hand, are primarily output layers which export information to other brain areas.

Anatomical characterization of the interplay between these reception and projection zones suggest that the cortex may be constructed of a continually repeating series of identical neural units called "modules." Each of these millions of modules may represent the most elemental information processing unit of the cortex.

Complex interconnections of modules are presumably required to produce the complicated analysis of biological signals necessary to support higher mental functions. Within sensory cortex cylindrical modules exist from surface to depth which respond to a particular type of sensory information presented in a specific area of the receptive surface of the external sensory receptors. In other words, a given module seems to be responsible for extracting information about the presence or absence of some particular stimulus feature in a restricted area of the sensory receptive field. This information, integrated with information from neighboring module about sensory activity in neighboring areas of the receptive field, may provide the basis for coherent perception of an environmental event. The extraction of single features and the subsequent recombination of this information has become the basic model for information processing cognitive psychology. Cognitions are thought to be composed of a series of individual features extracted singly and in

FIGURE 6

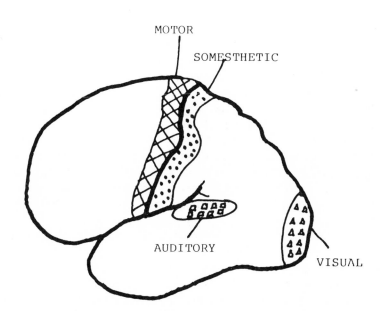

PRIMARY SENSORY AREAS OF THE CORTEX

combination from the sensory input channels and reassembled and organized into a coherent whole. If this idea actually represents the way in which information is processed, then the anatomical organization of the cerebral cortex is well suited to the task. The reader should be cautioned that the above is a simplification (and perhaps oversimplification) of the role of the cerebral cortex in cognitive function. Neurobiology is still a long way from a full understanding of this complex relationship.

THE PATHOBIOLOGY OF LEARNING AND COGNITIVE DISORDERS

In this final section we will attempt to examine what is known of the biological basis of some of the cognitive and learning disorders which are prevalent in children. The clinical literature very broadly categorizes childhood disorders into those which have defined organic basis and those which are considered to be "functional" disorders. The distinction is somewhat artificial since *all* disturbances of mental function must ultimately be the result of alterations in the ability of the brain processes to interact with the environment.

Disruptions of the information processing ability of the brain manifest themselves in disorders of; perception, orienting responses, memory, verbal expression, numeric ability, consciousness, attention, and personality. The biological manifestations of these disorders fall into three major categories; morphological alterations, electrophysiological alterations and biochemical alterations. The type and severity of the disorder is thought to be a function of both the amount of brain tissue affected and the specific location of the affected tissue within the brain.

An argument has raged in the field of neuropsychology about which of the two factors, the amount and severity of tissue damage or the specific location of the damage, is more important in determining the functional defects which result from injury to the brain. The former position is supported by the work of the Harvard psychologist Karl Lashley (1950) in the early 1950s using rodents. Lashley was concerned with searching for the pathways by which memories were laid down in the brain. To this end he affected the systematic destructions of multiple areas of the brain in order to observe the resulting effect on learning ability and retention. After nearly twenty years of investigations, Lashley concluded that the amount of tissue damage and the severity of the damage were the chief determinants of the type and magnitude of the functional losses observed. He speculated that the brain areas act in concert with one another as a functional mass and that any area is equally capable of performing a desired function. Small areas of damage produced little functional losses but large areas of damage, regardless of their location, produced severe learning deficits.

Lashley's findings did not agree completely with the earlier work of the French physician Pierre Paul Broca (1861). Broca was primarily interested in disorders of sensation and speech. He noted that a great preponderance of patients with speech disorders were later found to have significant tissue damage in one particular area of frontal lobe. The damage was almost invariably on the left side of the brain. Patients with similar damage in the same position on the opposite side of the brain, or patients with more severe damage elsewhere in the brain, did not exhibit these aberrations of speech. Thus the specific location of the damage seemed to be of prime importance in determining the resultant deficit. These two alternate ideas have remained unreconciled for decades. Current approaches to understanding brain damage, however, are attempting to integrate both of these views.

It has become popular in recent years to view the cerebral hemispheres as consisting of a system of primary, secondary and tertiary processing centers. These centers act in a coordinated fashion to process incoming sensory information. Primary sensory areas are responsible for reception of particular sensory information. Secondary areas are responsible for the organization of that sensory information into coherent images. Tertiary areas are thought to be responsible for integrating information from the sensory areas with other sensory modalities as well as with motor feedback information. Since these areas often lie adjacent to one another in the cerebral hemispheres, the type and severity of a disorder would be affected by both the location and the extent of a lesion.

Small lesions confined to the primary receiving area for vision will result in blindness. Lesions of the adjacent secondary visual area, which do not encompass the primary area, spare the ability to see but result in an inability to discriminate and recognize familiar objects (visual agnosia). More complex deficits are seen when brain lesions involve tertiary areas where sensory information from several systems converge. In these areas, complex integration of information all interact to produce higher mental functions such as spatial perception and calculation ability. Lesions of one such area of the frontal cortex produces a syndrome of "astereoagnosis," an inability to recognize objects by touch. Lesions of another such frontal area produces "acalulia" the inability to count or perform simple arithmetic calculations. The specific functions of the secondary and tertiary association areas is just beginning to be investigated.

Aside from gross anatomical or structural damage, neurobiologists are beginning to examine other indicators of dysfunction. Abnormal patterns of electrical activity in the EEG are currently being investigated as a possible diagnostic device for several types of disorders. Biochemical deficiencies have been observed in some brain disorders and have been able to be corrected pharmacologically. In this final section we will review some of the major childhood disorders and the electrophysiological, biochemical and anatomical substrates which underlie them.

Amentia

Amentia is defined clinically as retardation (IQ below 50) present before the age of eighteen. Its prevalence in the United States is nearly four children per thousand. The etiology of the disorder is varied and includes chromosomal aberrations, defective genoplasm development, perinatal complications and postnatal trauma. The anatomical manifestations come in the form of disordered development and organization of the cerebral cortex.

Normal cortical development depends on the critical timing of the production, migration and development of specific classes of neurons in specific layers of the six layered cortex. Disruption in any one of these processes could result in severe aberrations in both structure and connectivity in the adult brain. Anatomical investigations of cortical tissue in cases of amentia has revealed abnormal densities of neurons, particularly in the fourth cortical layer. We saw earlier that this is the major input layer to the altered distribution of neurons, investigators have observed marked changes in the general structure of individual neurons. The dendrites of cortical neurons throughout all layers were found to be thinner in their extent and lacking in certain structural features (dendritic spines) which are necessary for the establishment of normal synaptic contact with other neurons. It is not surprising that such a global disruption of neural organization manifests itself in such a profound perturbance of normal cognitive, perceptual and intellectual function.

Minimal Brain Dysfunction

The term minimal brain dysfunction (MBD) is used to classify children with impairments of learning not caused by inattentiveness, impairment of intelligence, or sociocultural mismatch. The disorder manifests itself in a variety of symptoms including, hyperactivity, disturbed conduct, reading difficulties, hyperemotionality and antisocial behavior. The definitions and classifications of the disorder are varied in the clinical literature, making any attempt at standardization of diagnosis difficult. Such standardizations are the first step toward the conduct of solid research. In their absence, it is difficult to make any generalizations from experimental data.

It has been reported that these children exhibit difficulties in the ability to process both visual and auditory information, a difficulty which often manifests itself in reading difficulties (dyslexia). Agnosias, or recognition disorders, are also common in these children, many of whom have difficulty recognizing both written words and visual symbols. Examinations of EEG have been carried out in recent years and have revealed some peculiarities of the EEG of MBD children.

Since the Label MBD is applied to a variety of conditions representing a variety of behavioral, intellectual, and perceptual problems it is difficult to establish criteria for including any given individual into the MBD classification. This difficulty severely hampers research in MBD. Most of the research that has been conducted has utilized children with specific learning disabilities (LD). LD children have been found to exhibit lower amplitude orienting responses which are correlated with decreased brain arousal. Analysis of *evoked potentials* has shown decreased amplitude of the later components of the *evoked response*. These components are thought to reflect integrative processing in the cortex. Expectancy waves were found to be diminished or absent in some dyslexics. Primary visual evoked responses in these children are also reduced. It should be noted that while some changes in brain

activity have been observed in some LD children, similar changes
do not appear in the majority of cases and their significance is thus
not clear.

Hyperkinesis

Hyperkinesis is characterized by a severe excess of motor activity and an attendant attentional deficit. The causal relationship between these two aspects of the disorder is unknown. Hyperkinetic
children are often disruptive in the classroom and can be prone to
episodic violence. It has been known for quite some time that the
symptom of overactivity in these children can be alleviated
through administration of drugs which, paradoxically, are brain
stimulants. Two brain stimulants amphetamine and methylpheni-
date are currently used with great success. The efficacy of these
compounds led some researchers to propose the source of hyperactivity in these children might in fact stem from a general deficiency in the physiological arousal of the brain. Their hyperactivity may be a constant attempt to increase stimulation. Peripheral
and central measures of arousal in hyperactive children have lent
some support to this theory. Measure of autonomic arousal such as
skin conductance and heart rate deceleration have been found to be
consistent with under-arousal in hyperactive children. Abnormalities of EEG records have been reported in 30-50% of hyperactive
children. Hyperactive children were found to display less beta activity in their EEG records and a general increase in slow wave
activity. Evoked response were found to be decreased in hyperactive kids. Both of these findings can be interpreted as indicative of under-arousal of the CNS. These facts coupled with the
efficacy of stimulant drugs in alleviating the symptoms tempt one
to conclude that hyperkinesis may be specifically an arousal problem.

Recently it has been shown that hyperactive children are deficient in one of the major neurotransmitters—dopamine. The relationship of this deficiency to attentional disorders is not clear. It is
interesting to note that one of the biochemical effects of those
drugs which have been found to be effective in the treatment in hyperkinesis is the increase of brain dopamine concentration. The effectiveness of these compounds may lie in their biochemical properties rather than their effect on brain excitability. Perhaps the real
truth lies in some combination of both factors.

Seizure Disorders

As originally defined by Englishman John Hughlings Jackson, (see Ref.) "epilepsy" refers to a disorder of consciousness and movement brought about by excessive and disordered neuronal discharges. Brain seizures result from paroxysmal neuronal discharges and result in transient disturbances in normal brain function. The prevalence of the disorder is estimated at nearly 0.5% in the United States.

The behavioral manifestations of brain seizures in children are quite varied including: convulsions, disorientation, confusion and in some cases uncontrolled violence. Seizure episodes in children tend to be less severe and shorter in duration than those of adults. Seizures can be classified into three broad categories: Grand mal, petit mal and psychomotor. Grand mal seizures are the most frequently observed in children and consist of several phases including: loss of consciousness, tonic stiffening of the body, clonic jerking of body musculature and post-convulsive sleep. Grand mal seizures are often precipitated by fever, fatigue or emotional stress. Petit mal seizures consist of a transient loss of consciousness with no attendant convulsions and normally last 5-10 seconds. Petit mal episodes are sometimes characterized as brief "absences." Recurrent bouts of petit mal seizures may mimic the appearance of mild retardation. The lapses of consciousness may be accompanied by a slight loss of body tone, facial twitches and lip smacking movements. Psychomotor seizures are manifested as transient alterations in behavior for which the patient is later amnesic, but during which the patient is capable of some limited interaction with the environment. These seizures are characterized by behavioral automatisms and severe thought disturbances including: disorientation, confusion and extreme agitation which can result in violent behavior. In some cases patients enter a fugue-like state during which they are able to perform customary activities but with no apparent conscious awareness.

All of the above types of seizure disorders are characterized electrophysiologically by the appearance of a specific abnormality of the EEG record known as the "spike/wave" complex (see Figure 7). The locus and origin of this abnormal neuronal discharge is varied and thought to be related to the type of behavioral disruption observed. Grand mal patients tend to show the most spike/wave activity in the frontal lobe of the cortex. In psychomo-

FIGURE 7

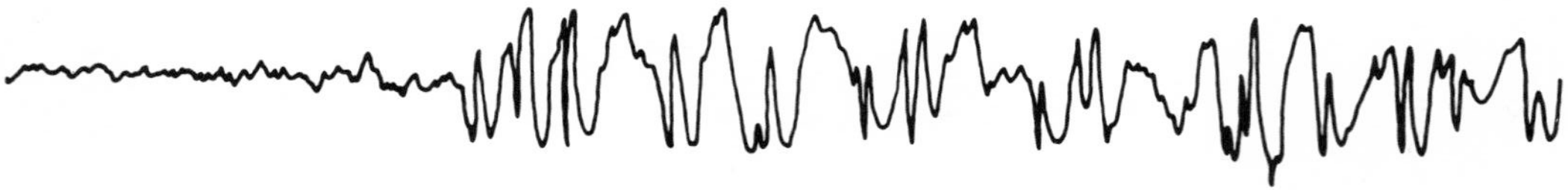

SPIKE AND WAVE COMPLEX FROM THE EEG OF A 6 YR. OLD EPILEPTIC BOY

tor patients spike/wave activity seem to be most pronounced in the temporal lobes. Spike/wave activity can be reduced by administration of certain anticonvulsive drugs. These compounds are currently used with great success to control the onset of seizures. Recently animal models of seizure disorders have been developed by producing abnormal spike/wave activity through injections of irritating chemicals into the brain. It is hoped that through the use of these models neurobiologists will gain further insight into the neural mechanisms which trigger the onset, spread and cessation of abnormal electrical activity in the brain.

SUMMARY

In the preceding pages we have attempted to examine some of the fundamental principles of neuroscience. We have reviewed some of what is known about the processes which subserve the functions of perception, cognition, learning and memory. As these are all areas of specific interest to educators, it is hoped that this brief overview has served to acquaint the reader with some of the important finds in the area of basic research. The basic mechanisms and principles which govern the operation of the complex biological network of our brain are as yet not fully understood. In part this is due to the immense complexity of the structure, as well as the difficulty of developing suitable animal models. What we hope to have shown in these pages, is something of the vulnerability of the brain to a variety of environmental interactions, and the role played by the resultant alterations in structure and function in some of the more prevalent cognitive disorders. It is not the intention of this brief review to serve as a "crash course" in basic neuroscience. Rather it is hoped that it has served to acquaint the reader with some of the constraints under which the neural machinery operates. Further we hope to have made relevant some of the current and important basic research findings. Continued research in the basic neural sciences will doubtless prove to be of great significance to educators in understanding the pathobiology of the disorders with which they are faced daily. Unraveling the "functional" nature of these disabilities was not an easy task for the field of education. The elucidation of the underlying neural mechanisms is expected to prove to be equally difficult. At this time we are only slightly closer to a complete understanding of these complex processes. It is hoped that future research will provide useful insights which will bring us closer to this final goal.

REFERENCES CITED

Blakemoor, C. and Cooper, G. F. Development of brain depends on visual experience. *Nature*, 1970, *228*, 477-478.

Broca, P. Remarques sur le siege de la faculté du langage Articule, suivies dune observation d'aphemie. *Society Anatomique de Paris, Bulletin et Memoire*, 1861, *6*, 330-357.

Jackson, J. H. in J. Taylor (ed.) Vol 1. *Selected writings of John Hughlings Jackson*. New York: Basic Books, 1958.

Kohler, I. The formation and transformation of the perceptual world. *Psychological Issues*, 1964, *3*, 1-173.

Lashley, K. S. In search of the engram. *Symposia of the Society for Experimental Biology*, 1950, *4*, 454-482.

Overton, D. A. State dependent or "Dissociated" learning procedures with pentobarbital. *JCPP*, 1964, *57*, 3-12.

SELECTED READINGS

Lindsay, P. H., & Norman, D. A. *Human information processing*. New York: Academic Press, 1977.

Posner, M. I. *Cognition: An introduction*. Glenview, IL. Scott, Forseman, 1973.

Melamed, L. E., & Forgus, R. *Perception: A cognitive-stage approach*. New York: McGraw Hill, 1976.

Taylor, E. Childhood Disorders. In H. M. Van Praag (Ed.), *Brain mechanisms and abnormal behavior (Part II)*. New York: Marcel Dekker Inc., 1980.

Pincus, J. H., & Tucker, G. J. *Behavioral neurology* (2nd Edition). New York: Oxford, 1978.

Denhoff, E., & Stern, L. *Minimal brain dysfunction: A developmental approach,* New York: Masson Pub., 1979.

Hemispheric Specialization and Functional Plasticity During Development

Susan Cohen Levine, PhD

ABSTRACT. Evidence from a variety of sources is reviewed suggesting that the cerebral hemispheres are specialized from birth or an early age. It is argued that findings of age differences in lateralization on certain tasks may be attributable to variations in the manner in which the tasks are carried out by subjects of different ages rather than to variations in the nature of the specialized processes of the cerebral hemispheres. Clinical observations of more rapid and complete recovery of function following brain injury in children than adults, therefore, cannot be explained in terms of an absence of hemispheric specialization early in life. Alternative explanations for this greater functional plasticity early in life are considered. Finally, misapplications and possible future applications of research findings on hemispheric specialization to educational practices are discussed.

HISTORICAL VIEW OF HEMISPHERIC SPECIALIZATION

Since Paul Broca's (1861) report to the French Anthropological Society that the loss of articulate speech typically follows injury to the left rather than the right cerebral hemisphere, the left cerebral hemisphere has been widely acknowledged as predominant for language functions. In fact, until relatively recently, the left hemisphere was regarded as dominant for all cognitive functions and the right hemisphere was relegated the title of "minor hemisphere." Despite the warnings of Hughlings Jackson in the 1870s (Jackson, 1958), it was not until the 1930s or later that large-scale

---

Susan Cohen Levine is an Associate Professor in the Departments of Pediatrics and Behavioral Sciences, University of Chicago, Chicago, IL 60637. Part of this paper was made possible by a grant from the Benton Fund.

77

studies of the deficits shown by patients with unilateral brain damage made it clear that the posterior portion of the right cerebral hemisphere is specialized for visuo-spatial functions (Weisenberg & McBride, 1935; Paterson & Zangwill, 1944).

Complementary Specialization

More recent research has continued to move us away from a theory of cerebral dominance to one of complementary specialization of the cerebral hemispheres. Evidence for complementary specialization of the hemispheres comes from a variety of sources: from studies of unilaterally brain damaged patients, from commissurotomy patients (patients in whom the corpus callosum, a massive nerve tract system connecting the cerebral hemispheres [see Figure 1] has been severed), and from studies of normal adults using lateralized input (Klein, Moscovitch, & Vigna, 1976; Sperry, 1974; Teuber, 1974; Levy, 1969; Kimura, 1967; Milner, 1960, 1968). (The use of lateralized input with normals depends upon the fact that each hemisphere receives sensory input primarily from the opposite side of the body and totally from the opposite visual field (see Figure 2).

It is now widely accepted that the left hemisphere is specialized for analytic, linguistic functions while the right hemisphere is specialized for more holistic visuo-spatial and tactuo-spatial functions as well as the perception of tonal patterns and environmental sounds. Such characterizations of the processes that are specialized to each hemisphere should only be regarded as primitive attempts to grasp the nature of hemispheric specialization. Moreover, these specializations are relative rather than absolute. We know that for all but the simplest cognitive tasks both hemispheres must be intact for optimal performance to be achieved. For example, it is known that patients with right cerebral injuries often have difficulty correctly producing and comprehending the prosodic information that accompanies speech, even though speech is typically regarded as a "left hemisphere function" (Tucker, Watson, & Heilman, 1977), while patients with left cerebral injuries frequently have difficulty perceiving and producing details in drawings, even though drawing is typically regarded as a "right hemisphere function" (Warrington, James, & Kinsbourne, 1966).

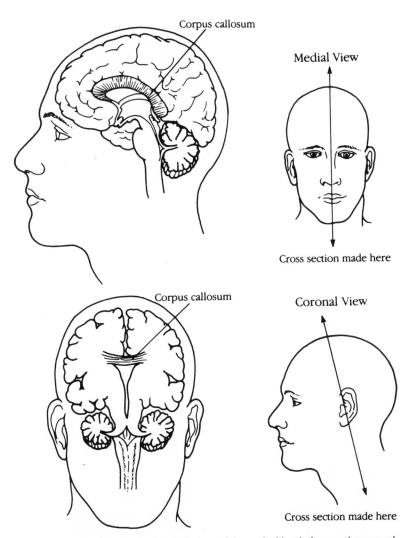

FIGURE 1. Sagittal (medial) and coronal views of the cerebral hemispheres and corpus callosum, the major nerve tract connecting the hemispheres. (From Springer, S. P., & Deutsch, G., *Left Brain, Right Brain*, p. 5. San Francisco: W. H. Freeman and Company, 1981. After Lindsay and Norman, *Human Information Processing*, p. 442, Academic Press, Inc., 1977). W. H. Freeman and Company, and Academic Press have granted permission to reprint this illustration.

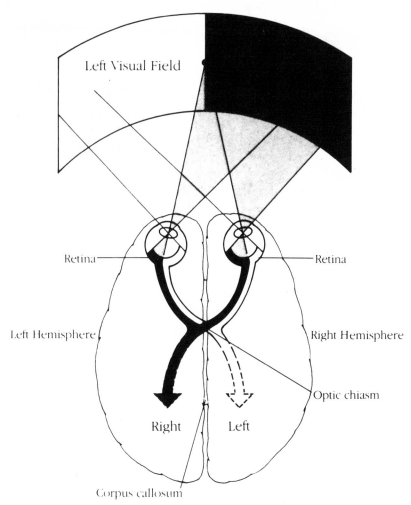

FIGURE 2. Information from the RVF is sent to visual cortex in the left hemisphere and information from the LVF is sent to visual cortex in the right hemisphere. This complete
crossover of visual information is a result of the way nerve fibers from the retina cross at the
optic chiasm. The visual areas of the two hemispheres normally communicate via the corpus
callosum. In commissurotomy patients, each hemisphere receives information from only
half the visual world if the eyes are kept from moving. (From Springer, S. P., & Deutsch,
G., *Left Brain, Right Brain,* p. 32. San Francisco: W. H. Freeman and Company, 1981).
W. H. Freeman and Company have granted permission to reprint this illustration.

DEVELOPMENTAL ISSUES IN HEMISPHERIC SPECIALIZATION

Studies on Brain-Damaged Children

There has been considerable interest in the development of adult patterns of complementary hemispheric specialization. Until recently, the cerebral hemispheres were regarded as being relatively unspecialized for some time during development, variously estimated to be from 5 to 11 years (Krashen, 1973; Lenneberg, 1967). This belief was based on two types of clinical findings with brain damaged children: (1) rapid recovery of language functions following injury to the left cerebral hemisphere in children (Lenneberg, 1967), implying that the right hemisphere might be able to take over language functions; (2) transient aphasia that occurs with nearly equal frequency following early brain injury to the left or right cerebral hemisphere (Basser, 1962).

More recent reports of childhood aphasia, reviewed by Woods and Teuber (1978), support the notion that children recover language functions more rapidly and completely than adults. While the capacity for recovery of function early in life is remarkable, however, it does have limitations. Dennis and Whitaker (1976) compared the language capacities of the left vs. right hemisphere in three 9-10-year-old children who had undergone surgical removal of one hemisphere before 5 months of age. Each of these children had Sturge-Weber-Dimitri syndrome, which results in gross abnormalities of the affected hemisphere. Two children with left hemisphere removal were compared to one with right hemisphere removal. While semantic and phonetic abilities were found to be similar in the three children, the two children with only a right hemisphere had significantly impaired syntactic abilities compared to the child with only a left hemisphere. For example, the children with only a right hemisphere (left hemidecorticates) showed little or no comprehension of complex syntactic forms such as passive sentences ("The car is pushed by the truck") while the child with only a left hemisphere (right hemidecorticate) was able to understand these sentences perfectly. (Normal children typically comprehend such passive sentences between the ages of 4 and 5 years.)

In a companion study (Kohn & Dennis, 1974), it was found that left hemidecorticates are superior to right hemidecorticates on visuo-spatial and route finding skills. In particular, the remaining left hemisphere of right hemidecorticates is only able to subsume those visuo-spatial functions that normally develop before age 10. Thus, while functional recovery following brain injury is greater in children than in adults, even in children, the originally specialized hemisphere is better able to carry out its functions than the opposite hemisphere. Moreover, when one cerebral hemisphere is injured early in life there is evidence that the overall IQ of the child suffers, and more so for larger than smaller lesions (Levine, Huttenlocher, & Duda, in preparation, ref. note 1). Thus, even early in life there is a price to be paid for the recovery of function (Teuber, 1974).

While Woods and Teuber (1978) support the notion that recovery of function following brain injury is more rapid and complete in children than adults, they refute the notion that aphasia follows left or right cerebral injury with nearly equal frequency early in life. In fact, in Woods and Teuber's (1978) series of children with unilateral brain damage, 25/34 with left hemisphere injuries had initial aphasic disturbances while only 4/31 with right hemisphere injuries (including two left-handers) had aphasic disturbances. The discrepancy between older and more recent reports on the frequency of aphasic disturbances following injury to the left vs. right cerebral hemisphere may be attributable to the introduction of antibiotics and mass immunizations. Prior to the use of these drugs, damage that was assumed to be isolated to the right hemisphere may in fact have been bilateral. This is particularly likely as many of the early cases of acquired aphasia in children arose as complications of systemic infectious diseases which without the benefit of modern medicine frequently resulted in diffuse encephalopathies.

In sum, findings of more rapid and complete recovery of language abilities following early brain injury support greater functional plasticity in children than in adults. This greater functional plasticity, however, is not attributable to a lack of hemispheric specialization in children, as was initially hypothesized by early investigators. Recent findings that aphasic symptoms typically follow injury to the left cerebral hemisphere in children indicate that hemispheric specialization is present in children. Alternative explanations for greater plasticity in children than adults have been proposed and will be discussed later in this paper.

These recent findings with brain damaged children are consistent with investigations of patterns of hemispheric specialization in normal children. At first glance, however, available developmental studies with normal children appear to provide conflicting information. Some of these studies report adult patterns of hemispheric specialization from infancy onwards (Entus, 1977; Kimura, 1963; Knox & Kimura, 1960; Liederman & Kinsbourne, 1980). In contrast, others report that specialization emerges over the course of development, with developmental changes occurring as late as puberty (Bryden, 1970; Lenneberg, 1967; Satz, Bakker, Teunissen, Goebel, & Van der Vlugt, 1975; Waber, 1976).

Studies on Normal Children

These apparently conflicting reports may be resolved by positing that developmental changes in hemispheric involvement reported for certain tasks are superimposed on an already existing foundation of hemispheric specialization. In fact, examination of the available experimental literature strongly suggests that the *foundations of hemispheric specialization are present from infancy, or even before.* First, anatomical evidence shows that the planum temporale, a region of the brain that is associated with language functions, is larger on the left than the right in infant and fetal brains as well as in adult brains (Geschwind & Levitsky, 1968; Wada, Clarke, & Hamm, 1975; Witelson & Pallie, 1973). Second, for both infants and adults electrophysiological studies show greater activity over the left hemisphere when speech sounds are presented, and over the right hemisphere when environmental sounds and musical stimuli are presented (Molfese, Freeman, & Palermo, 1975; Gardiner & Walter, 1977; Morgan, McDonald, & McDonald, 1971). Third, behavioral studies also provide support for the existence of hemispheric specialization in young infants. For example, several investigators have reported that young infants show rightward reflex, head turning, and directional looking-biases, most likely reflecting left hemisphere dominance over motor response systems (Siqueland & Lipsett, 1966; Turkewitz, Moreau, Davis, & Birch, 1969).

Recently, Liederman and Kinsbourne (1980) have reported that rightward head-turning biases are present only in infants with two right-handed parents. Infants with one left-handed parent showed no asymmetry, regardless of the sex of the left-handed parent, suggesting a genetic basis for hemispheric specialization. Moreover, dichotic listening techniques (involving simultaneous presentation of two different auditory stimuli, one to each ear) have revealed that infants as young as 22 days of age, the youngest tested, show a right-ear (left-hemisphere) advantage for the perception of speech sounds and a left-ear (right-hemisphere) advantage for the perception of musical tones.

Hemispheric Specialization and Cognitive Development

In view of these convincing findings that the cerebral hemispheres are specialized for at least some of their adult functions from birth onwards, what is the explanation(s) for studies that report changes in lateralization during development? As previously mentioned, it is possible that *hemispheric specialization for certain cognitive functions emerges later in development than hemispheric specialization for others.* Since studies of hemispheric specialization typically use only one task, it is possible that apparent inconsistencies in results are attributable to different developmental time courses of hemispheric specialization for the cognitive functions being tapped by different tasks. As Witelson (1977) points out, it is also possible that the emergence of lateralization on a particular task during development does not reflect a developmental change in hemispheric specialization. If the cognitive task under investigation is not yet in the child's repertoire (e.g., Witelson's example of speech production.) It is meaningless to consider the emergence of lateralization for that task at a later age as signaling the development of hemispheric specialization. Rather, each of the hemispheres may be specialized for particular cognitive processes from birth or an early age, and as the child develops a greater cognitive repertoire, each hemisphere may encompass more of the cognitive tasks that are optimally carried out by its processes. The distinction that is being drawn here is an important one. It involves viewing the emergence of lateralization on a particular cognitive task as reflecting a developmental change in hemispheric specialization vs. viewing the emergence of lateralization on a particular task as reflecting commitment of an already specialized hemisphere to that task.

Typically, investigators have interpreted the emergence of lateralization during development as signaling a developmental change in hemispheric specialization. The following examples illustrate that such interpretations may be erroneous.

1. Witelson (1976) reports a left-hand advantage for dichhaptic perception (bilateral tactile perception) of nonsense shapes by boys aged 6 to 14, but finds no hand asymmetry for girls in the same

age range. This finding was originally interpreted as suggesting that the right hemisphere is specialized for the spatial processes involved in this task from age 6 onwards for boys, while there is bilateral representation of this type of spatial processing at least until puberty for girls. In a later study, Witelson (personal communication, ref. note 2), found no hand asymmetry on this task for adults of either sex. The most parsimonious interpretation of this change in lateralization between age 14 and adulthood is that the information processes that adults are applying to this task are non-lateralized and different from those the male children are applying to this task, not that there is a change in hemispheric specialization. Of course, it would be possible to interpret the difference in laterality patterns shown by 6- to 14-year-old males vs. females in this same manner.

  2. Levine (in press) reports a LVF (left visual field)-right hemisphere advantage for the recognition of unfamiliar faces in children aged 10 and over but no lateral asymmetry on this task in 7-8-year-olds. In contrast, for the recognition of familiar, friends' faces, 7-8-year-olds, like adults, show a LVF-right hemisphere advantage. Interestingly, there is evidence that children under age 10 recognize previously unfamiliar faces in terms of salient, isolated features (bushy eyebrows), while children aged 10 and over recognize unfamiliar faces in terms of more configurational information (the ratio of the "distance from the hairline to the chin" to the "distance from the bridge of the nose to the upper lip") (Carey & Diamond, 1977; Diamond & Carey, 1977). In contrast, children as young as age 5, like older children and adults, are reported to recognize familiar faces in terms of configurational information (Diamond & Carey, 1977). Considered together, these findings suggest that the right hemisphere is differentially involved in the recognition of faces when faces are recognized in terms of configurational information. In fact, in certain situations adults recognize faces in terms of isolated features (e.g., when faces are inverted), and they show no lateral asymmetry (Yin, 1969; Leehey, Carey, Diamond, & Cahn, 1978). Thus, when subjects of any age recognize faces in terms of isolated features, the right hemisphere is not differentially involved in their recognition.

Information Processes and Hemispheric Specializations

  These two examples highlight the fact that one cannot ask which hemisphere is specialized for performing a particular task. Rather, one must identify the information processes for which each hemisphere is specialized and the information processes particular individuals use in carrying out specific tasks. This issue is particularly important in considering differences in laterality patterns between clinical populations and normals. For example, compared to normals, some dyslexic children show a decreased RVF-left hemisphere advantage for word recognition (Marcel, Katz, & Smith, 1974). This may be attributable to differences in the information processes that normals and dyslexics apply to reading, rather than to underlying group differences in hemispheric specialization. In particular, these dyslexic children may take a more spatial, less phonetic approach to word recognition than normals, thereby decreasing left hemisphere involvement in this task. Normals might show the same laterality pattern for word recognition as dyslexics if they applied the same information processes to this task. It is very important to realize that the same cognitive task may involve different information processes for people who differ in age, sex, and overall ability level.

INDIVIDUAL DIFFERENCES IN HEMISPHERIC SPECIALIZATION

Handedness

This brings us to the topic of individual differences in hemispheric specialization. It is widely accepted that there are group differences in patterns of hemispheric specialization between right-handed individuals (dextrals) and left-handed individuals (sinistrals) (Rasmussen & Milner, 1973); Hecaen & Sauget, 1971) and males and females (McGlone, 1980; Harris, 1978). Typically, the cerebral hemispheres of sinistrals and females are regarded as being more bilaterally organized than the hemispheres of dextrals and males. Thus, reports in the literature suggest that sinistrals (Rasmussen & Milner, 1971) and females (McGlone, 1980) are less likely to experience aphasic symptoms and are more likely to recover language functions than dextrals following left hemisphere injury. In addition, even strongly right-handed individuals with left-handed relatives are more likely to recover from the aphasic disturbances that follow left hemisphere injury than strongly right-handed subjects with no left-handed relatives (Luria, 1970).

While it has commonly been assumed that dextrals are homogeneous in their lateralization for cognitive functions, recently it has been realized that even dextrals of the same sex may differ in their patterns of hemispheric involvement in cognitive tasks. Evidence from brain damaged patients suggests that the left hemisphere subserves language functions in the vast majority of dextrals (95% or more). In contrast to this, only about 70% of normal dextrals show the expected laterality patterns for processing verbal stimuli or visuo-spatial stimuli on standard laterality tasks. The discrepancy between these laterality findings and assumed homogeneity in patterns of hemispheric specialization among dextrals has typically been attributed to random error in the measurements used (Teng, 1981) or to subjects' perceptual biases (directional scanning preferences induced by reading habits) (White, 1969). Neither of these explanations, however, adequately accounts for the large variations in direction or degree of lateralization among dextrals on verbal and spatial laterality tasks.

Hemispheric Arousal Asymmetry and Hemispheric Specialization

Levy, Heller, Banich, and Burton (1983) suggest an alternative explanation for this apparent discrepancy. Integrating the evidence from brain damaged patients and normals, they hypothesize that dextrals are homogeneous in underlying hemispheric specialization, but that they differ in direction and degree of characteristic arousal asymmetry of the two hemispheres. That is, while the left cerebral hemisphere is specialized for verbal-analytic functions and the right hemisphere for spatial-Gestalt functions in virtually all dextrals, the left hemisphere is characteristically more aroused than the right hemisphere in some dextrals and the right hemisphere is characteristically more aroused than the left hemisphere in others. These individual variations in hemispheric arousal asymmetry are superimposed on hemispheric specialization so as to decrease left hemisphere participation in verbal tasks in individuals with arousal asymmetries in favor of the right hemisphere and to decrease right hemisphere participation in spatial tasks in individuals with arousal asymmetries in favor of the left hemisphere.

Levy et al. (1983) review evidence from a variety of sources suggesting that dextrals differ in hemispheric arousal asymmetry, e.g., measurement of EEG asymmetries (Furst, 1976; Ray, Newcombe, Semon, & Cole, 1981); measurement of cerebral blood flow asymmetries (Gur & Reivich, 1980); and measurement of the direction of conjugate lateral eye movements to reflective questions (Bakan, 1969; Gur, Gur, & Harris, 1975). In agreement with these findings, Levy et al. (1983) found that individuals with greater left hemisphere involvement in a nonsense syllable identification task show less right hemisphere involvement in a free vision face processing task in which subjects judged the intensity of emotional expression on faces, while individuals with less left hemisphere participation in the nonsense syllable task show greater right hemisphere participation in the face processing task. The results of this study suggest that *certain dextrals rely more on right hemisphere processing while others rely more on left hemisphere processing on verbal as well as spatial tasks, possibly because of individual variations in characteristic hemispheric arousal asymmetry.*

Levine, Banich, and Koch-Weser (submitted ref. note 3), reasoned that individual dextrals' laterality scores on a task that is non-lateralized for the group of dextrals as a whole might index characteristic arousal asymmetry. In fact, they found that subjects with a left visual field-right hemisphere bias on a chair recognition task, a task non-lateralized for the group as a whole, show a highly significant left visual field-right hemisphere advantage for the recognition of visuo-spatial stimuli such as faces, houses, and cars. In contrast, dextrals who show a left hemisphere bias on chair recognition show a non-significant advantage in favor of the right hemisphere in the recognition of the other classes of visuo-spatial stimuli (see Figure 3).

Existence of Hemispheric Arousal Asymmetries

Existing evidence suggests that hemispheric arousal asymmetries are characteristic of individuals as they are related to a variety of stable cognitive and personality measures (Gur & Reivich, 1980; Gur & Gur, 1975). For example, Gur and Reivich (1980) report that dextrals with asymmetric right hemisphere blood flow perform better on a spatial, Gestalt completion test than dextrals with asymmetric left hemisphere blood flow (asymmetric hemispheric blood flow is considered an accurate index of relative metabolic rate of each hemisphere). Individual variations in characteristic arousal asymmetry of the cerebral hemispheres have not yet

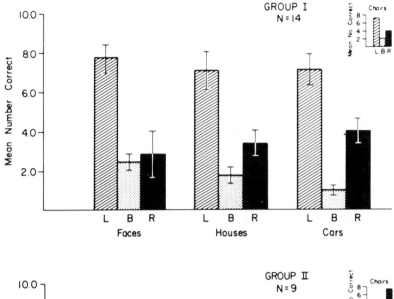

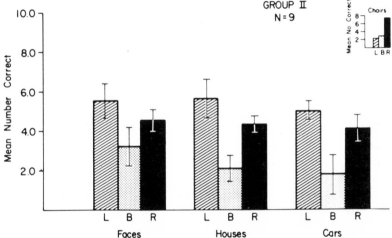

FIGURE 3. (a) Mean number of correct LVF (L), Bilateral (B), and RVF (R) trials for faces, houses, and cars for Group I (subjects with better recognition of chairs in the LVF, N = 14). (b) Mean number of correct LVR (L), Bilateral (B), and RVF (R) trials for faces, houses, and cars for Group II (subjects with better recognition of chairs in the RVF, N = 9). (From Levine, S. C., Banich, M. T., & Koch-Weser, M., Variations in patterns of cerebral asymmetry among dextrals. Submitted for publication, 1983.)

been explored in developmental studies. *It is an interesting question whether these arousal asymmetries are innate, or are influenced by an individual's early experience, interests, abilities, and/or by maturational changes in the brain.*

DEVELOPMENTAL CHANGES IN BRAIN ORGANIZATION: POSSIBLE EXPLANATIONS FOR DEVELOPMENTAL CHANGES IN FUNCTIONAL PLASTICITY

Findings from studies of unilaterally brain damaged children and from studies of normal infants and children suggest that the foundations of hemispheric specialization are present very early in life. However, these findings should *not* be interpreted as evidence that there are no developmental changes in brain organization during development. In fact, the finding that children are better able to recover functions following brain injury (functional plasticity) than adults requires that one posit some organizational changes in the brain.

Developmental Brain Changes

One major change in the brain during development involves *myelinization* of the corpus callosum, the massive fiber system that connects the two hemispheres. *Myelin,* a fatty sheath that covers nerve fibers, is extremely important in the speed of neural transmission. Anatomical studies show that myelinization of the callosum is a slow process, not beginning until about one year of age and not complete until age 10 or later (Yakovlev & Lecours, 1967). Thus, the anatomical picture of the corpus callosum changes radically during the first decade of life. In an electrophysiological study, Salamy (1978) has shown that the latency difference between ipsilateral (same side) and contralateral (opposite side) cortical evoked response to tactile stimulation of the index finger decreases with median log age between ages 3-½ and 10. This decrease in latency difference between contralateral and ipsilateral evoked response may be attributable to increasing ability of the corpus callosum to transmit tactile information to the hemisphere that is ipsilateral to the finger that is touched (Salamy, 1978). Supporting this hypothesis, the time course of the latency change is in striking agreement with the time course of myelinization of the corpus callosum. In a behavioral study, Galin, Johnstone, Nakell, and Herron (1979) have demonstrated that the advantage of same hand over different hand judgments of whether two pieces of cloth are the same or different in texture decreases between the ages of 3 and 5 years (older children were not tested). Presumably, this reflects increased functional communication between the hemispheres during development, which in turn reflects development of the corpus callosum.

The development of the corpus callosum provides a viable explanation for the greater functional plasticity of the child's brain than the adult's brain. Levy (in press) hypothesizes that each hemisphere initially has a primary program of specialization, and a secondary program that includes the specialized processes of the opposite hemisphere. During the course of normal development, each hemisphere's primary program of specialization becomes elaborated, while the secondary program of specialization is suppressed. Presumably these changes depend upon the development of the corpus callosum and upon normal input from the opposite hemisphere. Evidence for this is as follows. First, in cases of agenesis of the corpus callosum (congenital absence of the corpus callosum), the hemispheres are more bilaterally organized than normal (Netley, 1977). It is possible that this bilateralization of function is affected by the absence of the regulatory functions of the corpus callosum. Second, following hemispherectomy early in life, both the primary and secondary programs of the remaining hemisphere become elaborated (Dennis & Whitaker, 1976). Interestingly, this dramatic plasticity is not evident in adult hemispherectomy patients, presumably because the secondary programs of each hemisphere have already been suppressed (Smith, 1966). The immaturity of the corpus callosum during the first decade of life may result in the secondary programs of each hemisphere being preserved, allowing for more rapid and complete recovery of function following brain injury than is possible later in life.

A different approach to the plasticity issue has been taken by other investigators. Huttenlocher, de Counter, Garey, and Van der Loos (1982) suggest that redundant neural connections present early in development may impart plasticity to the developing nervous system. Huttenlocher (1979) and Huttenlocher et al. (1982) report a period of rapid increase in synaptic density up until about age one (when synaptic density is 50-60% above the adult value), followed by a period of gradual synaptic elimination between ages one and adolescence in the middle frontal gyrus and area 17 of the visual cortex, respectively (see Figure 4). If this proliferation of connections during early development is related to functional plasticity, then recovery from injury or dysfunction (1) should be greatest during the period when the number of synapses is high, and (2) might lead to persistence of synapses that would normally

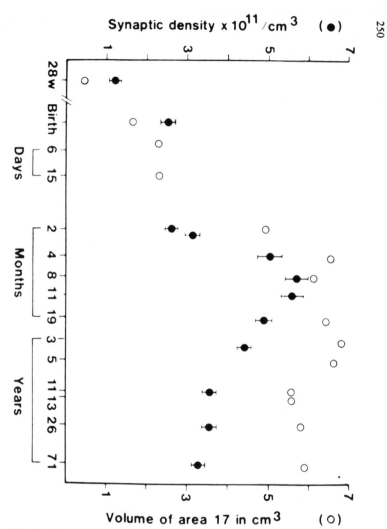

FIGURE 4. Mean synaptic density values for all layers of area 17 (visual cortex) are indicated by the closed circles (left-hand scale). Each point represents the mean of several thousand counts. Vertical bars represent standard errors of 6 separate synapse counts in the same brain in strips of cortex 3 μm in width. The open circles (right-hand scale) plot mean volume of area 17. Age is plotted on a logarithmic scale. (From Huttenlocher, P. R., de Courten, C., Gorey, L. J., & Van der Loos, H., Synaptogenesis in human visual cortex—evidence for synapse elimination during normal development. *Neuroscience Letters*, 1982, *33*, p. 250.)

be eliminated. There is evidence for both (1) and (2) with respect to the visual cortex. First, in the young child loss of fixation due to a strabismic eye can readily be reversed by patching the normal eye until about 18 months of age, with an upper limit of 5-7 years (Assaf, 1982). It is tantalizing that the time course of this plasticity resembles that of synaptic elimination in the human visual cortex. Second, anatomic evidence from congenitally strabismic Siamese cats supports the persistence of connections that would otherwise disappear. It is possible that the persistence of these connections helps compensate for the effects of abnormal visual input (Shatz, 1977). Similar effects may account for the sparing of language functions following early insult to the left cerebral hemisphere.

We are left with two viable, not mutually exclusive, hypotheses for functional plasticity early in life—the presence of a relatively undeveloped corpus callosum and the proliferation of synaptic connections. *The young brain has apparently evolved to handle complex information, in view of evidence that specialized cerebral hemispheres are present from birth. At the same time, the young brain has apparently evolved certain safety factors that protect it from what otherwise could be devastating effects of early brain injuries.*

HEMISPHERIC SPECIALIZATION AS AN EDUCATIONAL METAPHOR

Recently, educational journals have devoted a great amount of attention to the implications of hemispheric specialization for educational practices (see *Current Index to Journals in Education* for references). These publications have primarily admonished educators for not teaching the right hemisphere. Typical "left hemisphere" teaching practices have been held responsible for children's deficiencies in such wide-ranging non-verbal skills as map-reading, constructional abilities, musical abilities, artistic abilities, creativity, etc. (Bogen, 1978; Prince, 1978).

It is certainly the case that our educational system has paid relatively more attention to the development of verbal than of non-verbal skills. Depending upon one's viewpoint, this may or may not be desirable. However, restating this fact in terms of hemispheric specialization, i.e., that we are educating the left and not the right side of the brain, merely serves as an inappropriate metaphor, and confuses the issue.

Holistic Approach

The scientific study of hemispheric specialization does not provide any simple formula for assigning such complex disciplines as art or music to one side of the brain or the other. Rather, as previously discussed in this article, research on hemispheric specialization indicates that we are *whole-brained creatures,* and that all but the simplest tasks require the *integration of processes of both cerebral hemispheres.* Examination of the abilities of commissurotomy patients provides convincing evidence that on complex tasks requiring sustained attention, an isolated hemisphere—even the hemisphere that is specialized for a particular task—is not nearly as competent as an intact brain (Levy, in press).

In addition to the theoretical problems involved in attempting to educate one cerebral hemisphere vs. the other, the practical issues of how one would go about doing this are not trivial. We are not, after all, educating commissurotomy patients. Recent publications seem to be suggesting that more non-verbal, artistic stimulation be introduced, and perhaps our educational system needs this change. It is unnecessary, and at best inaccurate, however, to couch these recommendations in terms of educating the right hemisphere.

The above comments should not be interpreted to mean that there are no possible educational implications of research on hemispheric asymmetries. For example, findings that some individuals have a relatively more aroused right hemisphere while others have a relatively more aroused left hemisphere, and that these arousal patterns are associated with specific ability and personality patterns, might guide the way we instruct individual students. An interesting research question is whether asymmetric arousal patterns that are present early in life might be shifted in one direction or the other based on specific early experiences. Such applications of research on hemispheric asymmetries to educational practices must await sufficient experimental exploration. However tantalizing current research findings may be, it is important to bear in mind that the study of *hemispheric specialization is a young science* that has not yet reached a point where specific educational applications of research findings can be made.

REFERENCE NOTES

1. Levine, S. C., Huttenlocher, P. R., & Duda, G. Cognitive functioning in relation to CAT-scan findings in hemiplegic children. In preparation.
2. Witelson, S. Personal communication.
3. Levine, S., Banich, M. T., & Koch-Weser, M. Variations in patterns of lateral asymmetry among dextrals. Submitted for publication, 1983.

REFERENCES

Assaf, A. A. The sensitive period: Transfer of fixation after occulsion for strabismic amblyopia. *British Journal of Ophthalmology*, 1982, *66*, 64-70.

Bakan, P. Hypnotizability, laterality of eye movements and functional brain asymmetry. *Perceptual and Motor Skills*, 1969, *28*, 927-932.

Basser, L. S. Hemiplegia of early onset and the faculty of speech with special reference to the effects of hemispherectomy. *Brain*, 1962, *85*, 427-460.

Bogen, J. E. The other side of the brain. VII: Some educational aspects of hemispheric specialization. *UCLA Educator*, 1975, *17*, 24-32.

Broca, P. Sur la siège de la faculté de language articulé avec deux observations d'aphemie (perte de parole). Paris, 1891.

Bryden, M. P. Laterality effects in dichotic listening: Relations with handedness and reading ability in children. *Neuropsychologia*, 1970, *8*, 443-450.

Carey, S., & Diamond, R. From piecemeal to configurational representation of faces. *Science*, 1977, *195*, 312-314.

Dennis, M., & Whitaker, H. A. Language acquisition following hemidecortication: Linguistic superiority of the left over the right hemisphere. *Brain and Language*, 1976, *3*, 404-433.

Diamond, R., & Carey, S. Developmental changes in the representation of faces. *Journal of Experimental Child Psychology*, 1977, *23*, 1-22.

Entes, A. K. Hemispheric asymmetry in processing of dichotically presented speech and non-speech stimuli by infants. In A. J. Segalowitz & F. A. Gruber (Eds.), *Language development and neurological theory*. New York: Academic Press, 1977.

Furst, C. J. EEG asymmetry and visuospatial performance. *Nature*, 1976, *260*, 254-255.

Galin, D., Johnstone, J., Nakell, L., & Herron, J. Development of the capacity for tactile information transfer between hemispheres in normal children. *Science*, 1979, *204*, 1330-1331.

Gardiner, M. F., & Walter, D. O. Evidence of hemispheric specialization from EEG. In S. Harnod, R. W. Doty, L. Goldstein, J. Jaynes, & G. Krauthamer (Eds.), *Lateralization in the nervous system*. New York: Academic Press, 1977.

Geschwind, N., & Levitsky, W. Human brain: Left-right asymmetries in temporal speech region. *Science*, 1968, *161*, 186-187.

Gur, R. E., & Gur, R. C. Defense mechanisms, psychosomatic symptomatology, and conjugate lateral eye movements. *Journal of Consulting and Clinical Psychology*, 1975, *43*, 416-420.

Gur, R. E., Gur, E. C., & Harris, L. J. Cerebral activation, as measured by subjects' lateral eye movements, is influenced by experimenter location. *Neuropsychologia*, 1975, *13*, 35-44.

Gur, R. C., & Reivich, M. Cognitive task effects on hemispheric blood flow in humans: Evidence for individual differences in hemispheric activation. *Brain and Language*, 1980, *9*, 78-92.

Harris, L. J. Sex differences in spatial ability: Possible environmental, genetic, and neurological factors. In M. Kinsbourne (Ed.), Asymmetrical function of the brain. Cambridge: Cambridge University Press, 1978.

Hecaen, H., & Sauget, J. Cerebral dominance in left-handed subjects. Cortex, 1971, 7, 19-48.

Huttenlocher, P. R. Synaptic density in human frontal cortex: Developmental changes and effects of aging. Brain Research, 1979, 163, 195-205.

Huttenlocher, P. R., de Courten, C., Garey, L. J., & Van der Loos, H. Synaptogenesis in human visual cortex—evidence for synapse elimination during normal development. Neuroscience Letters, 1982, 33, 247-252.

Jackson, J. H. Selected writings of John Hughlings Jackson (J. Taylor, Ed.). New York: Basic Books, 1958.

Kimura, D. Speech lateralization in young children as determined by an auditory test. Journal of Comparative and Physiological Psychology, 1963, 56, 899-902.

Kimura, D. Functional asymmetry of the brain in dichotic listening. Cortex, 1967, 3, 163-178.

Klein, P., Moscovitch, M., & Vigna, C. Perceptual asymmetries and attentional mechanisms in tachistoscopic recognition of words and faces. Neuropsychologia, 1976, 14, 44-66.

Knox, C., & Kimura, D. Cerebral processing of nonverbal sounds in boys and girls. Neuropsychologia, 1970, 8, 227-237.

Kohn, B., & Dennis, M. Selective impairments of visuo-spatial abilities in infantile hemiplegics after right cerebral hemidecortication. Neuropsychologia, 1974, 12, 505-512.

Krashen, S. Laterlization, language learning, and the critical period. Language Learning, 1973, 23, 63-74.

Leehey, S. C., Carey, S., Diamond, R., & Cahn, A. Upright and inverted faces: The right hemisphere knows the difference. Cortex, 1978, 14, 411-419.

Lenneberg, E. Biological foundations of language. New York: John Wiley and Sons, 1967.

Levine, S. Developmental changes in right hemisphere involvement in face recognition. In C. T. Best (Ed.), Developmental neuropsychology and education: Hemispheric specialization and integration. New York: Academic Press, in press.

Levy, J. Possible basis for the evolution of lateral specialization of the human brain. Nature, 1969, 224, 614-615.

Levy, J. Interhemispheric collaboration: Single-mindedness in the asymmetric brain. In C. T. Best (Ed.), Developmental neuropsychology and education: Hemispheric specialization and integration. New York: Academic Press, in press.

Levy, J., Heller, W., Banich, M. T., & Burton, L. A. Are variations among right-handed individuals in perceptual asymmetries caused by characteristic arousal differences between hemispheres? Journal of Experimental Psychology: Human Perception and Performance, 1983, 9, 329-359.

Liederman, J., & Kinsbourne, M. Rightward motor bias in newborns depends upon parental right-handedness. Neuropsychologia, 1980, 18, 579-584.

Luria, G. R. Traumatic aphasia. The Hague: Mouton, 1970.

Marcel, T., Katz, L., & Smith, M. Laterality and reading proficiency. Neuropsychologia, 1974, 12, 131-139.

McGlone, J. Sex differences in human brain asymmetry: A critical survey. The Brain and Behavioral Sciences, 1980, 3, 218-263.

Milner, B. Impairment of visual recognition and recall after right temporal lobectomy in man. Paper presented at Psychonomic Society Meeting, Chicago, 1960.

Milner, B. Visual recognition and recall after right temporal lobe excision in man. Neuropsychologia, 1968, 6, 191-209.

Molfese, D., Freeman, R., & Palermo, D. The ontogeny of brain lateralization for speech and non-speech stimuli. Brain and Language, 1975, 2, 356-368.

Morgan, A. H., McDonald, P. J., & McDonald, H. Differences in bilateral alpha activity as a function of experimental task, with a note on lateral eye movements and hypnotizability. *Neuropsychologia*, 1971, *9*, 459-469.

Netley, C. Dichotic listening of callosal agenesis and Turner's Syndrome patients. In S. J. Segalowitz & F. A. Gruber (Eds.), *Language development and neurological theory.* New York: Academic Press, 1977.

Paterson, A., & Zangwill, O. Disorders of visual space perception associated with lesions of the right cerebral hemisphere. *Brain*, 1944, *64*, 331-358.

Prince, G. Putting the other half of the brain to work. *Training: The Magazine of Human Resources Development*, 1978, *15*, 57-61.

Rasmussen, T., & Milner, B. The role of early left-brain injury in determining lateralization of cerebral speech functions. In S. J. Dimond & D. A. Blizard (Eds.), *Evolution and lateralization of the brain. Annals of the New York Academy of Sciences.* New York: New York Academy of Sciences, 1973.

Ray, W. J., Newcombe, N., Semon, J., & Cole, P. M. Spatial abilities, sex differences and EEG functioning. *Neuropsychologia*, 1981, *19*, 719-722.

Salamy, A. Commissural transmission: Maturational changes in humans. *Science*, 1978, *200*, 1409-1441.

Satz, P., Bakker, P. J., Teunissen, J., Goebel, R., & Van der Vlugt, H. Developmental parameters of the ear asymmetry: A multivariate approach. *Brain and Language*, 1975, *2*, 171-185.

Shatz, C. J. Anatomy of interhemispheric connections in the visual system of Boston siamese and ordinary cats. *Journal of Comparative Neurology*, 1977, *173*, 497-518.

Siqueland, E. R., & Lippsett, L. P. Conditioned head-turning in human newborns. *Journal of Experimental Child Psychology*, 1966, *4*, 366-377.

Smith, A. Speech and other functions after left (dominant) hemispherectomy. *Journal of Neurology, Neurosurgery, and Psychiatry*, 1966, *29*, 467-471.

Sperry, R. W. Lateral specialization in the surgically separated hemispheres. In P. J. Vinken and G. W. Bruyn (Eds), *The neurosciences: Third study program.* Cambridge, MA: M.I.T. Press, 1974.

Teng, E. L. Dichotic ear difference is a poor index for the functional asymmetry between the cerebral hemispheres. *Neuropsychologia*, 1981, *19*, 235-240.

Teuber, H. L. Why two brains? In F. O. Schmitt & F. J. Worden (Eds.), *The neurosciences: Third study program.* Cambridge, MA: M.I.T. Press, 1974.

Tucker, R. M., Watson, R. T., & Heilman, K. Discrimination and evocation of affectively intoned speech in patients with right parietal disease. *Neurology*, 1977, *27*, 947-950.

Turkewitz, G., Moreau, T., Davis, L., & Birch, H. Factors affecting lateral differentiation in the human newborn. *Journal of Experimental Child Psychology*, 1969, *8*, 483-493.

Waber, D. P. Sex differences in cognition: A function of maturation rate? *Science*, 1976, *192*, 572-574.

Wada, J. A., Clarke, R., & Hamm, A. Cerebral hemispheric asymmetry in humans: Cortical speech zones in 100 adults and 100 infant brains. *Archives of Neurology*, 1975, *32*, 239-246.

Warrington, E. K., James, M., & Kinsbourne, M. Drawing disability in relation to laterality of cerebral lesion. *Brain*, 1966, *89*, 53-82.

Weisenberg, T., & McBride, K. E. *Aphasia: A clinical and psychological study.* New York: Commonwealth Fund, 1935.

White, M. Laterality difference in perception: A review. *Psychological Bulletin*, 1969, *72*, 382-405.

Witelson, S. F. Sex and the single hemisphere. *Science*, 1976, *193*, 425-427.

Witelson, S. F. Early hemisphere specialization and interhemisphere plasticity: An empirical and theoretical review. In S. J. Segalowitz & F. A. Gruber (Eds.), *Language development and neurological theory.* New York: Academic Press, 1977.

Witelson, S. F., & Pallie, W. Left hemisphere specialization for language in the newborn: Neuroanatomical evidence of asymmetry. *Brain*, 1973, *96*, 641-647.

Woods, B. T., & Teuber, H. L. Changing patterns of childhood aphasia. *Annals of Neurology*, 1978, *3*, 273-280.

Yakovlev, P., & Lecours, A. The meylogenetic cycle of regional maturation of the brain. In A. Minkowski (Ed.), *Regional development of the brain in early life*. Oxford: Blackwell Scientific Publications, 1967.

Yin, R. K. Looking at upside-down faces. *Journal of Experimental Psychology*, 1969, *81*, 141-147.

Cognitive Levels Matching:
An Instructional Model and a Model
of Teacher Change

Patricia Kennedy Arlin, PhD

ABSTRACT. Cognitive levels matching refers to a teacher's ability to use formal and informal means of assessing the cognitive levels of students and to adapt instruction according to student needs. This ability is contingent upon the teacher acquiring a "developmental perspective." The methods for acquiring this perspective suggest a fundamental change in the way the teacher thinks about instruction. The renewed emphasis on cognitive levels matching is the result of current interest in neurobiological research, particularly that of Epstein. Although cognitive levels matching (CLM) cannot directly test his hypotheses, the emphasis of CLM has become an emphasis on strategies to assist teachers to teach from a developmental point-of-view. Four informal strategies are described which can assist teachers to teach "from the child's point-of-view and thus to begin the process of matching."

COGNITIVE LEVEL MATCHING

In the early 1960s, J. McVicker Hunt described the major problem facing education as "the problem of the match" (1962). While the framework for cognitive levels matching has thus been in place

Patricia Arlin, Department of Educational Psychology, The University of British Columbia, 2125 Main Mall, Vancouver, B. C. V6T 125, Canada.

for a number of years, what was required was the provision of techniques for acquiring a developmental perspective, the actual specification of educational needs in terms of stages or levels, and developmentally informed means of evaluating instructional materials in terms of intellectual ability and developmental readiness. Cognitive Levels Matching provides a means of fulfilling these requirements. It provides a framework for both curriculum development and a developmental curriculum. And the process becomes a model of teacher change.

Cognitive levels are defined primarily in terms of Piaget's four stages of development (Arlin, reference note 1; Brooks, Fusco, Grennon, 1983; Epstein, 1981). The term levels is used instead of stages because Inhelder and Piaget (1958) employ this term to describe the performance of children and adolescents on a variety of formal reasoning tasks; characterizing trial and error approaches of young children to the solution of problems as Level IA and the sophisticated use of various logic forms and concepts as Level IIIB.

Inhelder and Piaget's description of six levels roughly approximates three of their stages in the development of logical thinking: preoperational, concrete operational thought and formal operational thought. Figure 1 is a summary of these stages with the major cognitive conquest of each stage as characterized by Elkind (1967). The broad outline of Piaget's model is a familiar one but it is important to emphasize that each cognitive conquest associated with each stage represents a "new means" which becomes available to the child for actively building up knowledge of the world. For example is the baby's own action on objects that is the basis for knowledge in the sensorimotor stage. The young child uses symbol or language as a way of learning about objects so that not only her actions but also her words, sounds, and actions are constructed about and between objects through language. Each of these new ways of constructing knowledge suggests strengths and limitations in child thought and reinforces the basic Piagetian notion that child thought really is different in kind than adult thought. The child's point-of-view, the child's construction of knowledge, is different than the teacher's.

The current popularity of the concept of cognitive levels matching is due in large measure to the neurobiological research and speculations about the educational implications of that research by Epstein (1974a, 1974b, 1978, 1981). His brain growth periodicity proposals are offered as the neurobiological basis for stage transitions and change of level in cognitive development.

BRAIN GROWTH STAGES	"COGNITIVE LEVELS"	PIAGET'S STAGES
3-10 months Neuron development cerebelium		1. Sensorimotor (0-18 months) -Object-
2-4 Years angular gyrus Hearing/binocular vision language development	IA - Play IB - Trial/Error	2. Preoperational (2 - (5-7) yrs.) -Symbol-
6-8 Years angular gyrus reading/writing	IIA - Some attempt at system IIB - systematic but does not generalize	3. Concrete Operations ((5-7) - (11-14) or 15-17 or ?) -Classify- -Seriate- -Conserve-
10-12 Years rear right hemisphere prefrontal cortex abstract thought and problem solving	IIIA - Systematic, generalizes, but doesn't exhaust possibilities	4. Formal Operations (11-14 Years or?) -Thought Itself-
14-16 Years angular gyrus (?) rear left hemisphere problem finding and self-awareness	IIIB - fully formal, considers rival hypotheses etc.	5. Post-Formal (15-17 or ?) -Frameworks-

FIGURE 1. Brain growth stages, cognitive developmental stages and cognitive levels. Brain growth stages were developed by Epstein and Sylwester; cognitive levels were developed by Arlin; and Piaget's Stages were developed by Piaget (Elkind, 1969).

They are reinforced by the remarkable parallel between the ages of significant brain growth and the ages of potential onset of new cognitive stages as illustrated in the figure above. The original working hypothesis of the CLM projects was:

If neurobiological changes occur on a regular timetable that parallels that specified by Piaget for the onset of the stages of cognitive development then these neurobiological changes may bring about a structural change in the brain which may set up the possibility that a change in cognitive functioning may occur. The Piagetian model represents a first approximation of what those functional changes might entail. Particularly at the onset of the stage of formal operations. It is hypothesized that those functional changes will only occur in the presence of appropriate instructional intervention and experience and not outside these conditions.

While Epstein's neurobiological research and his related educational hypotheses were the initial impetus for the CLM projects, it is clear that such projects cannot provide a direct test of these hypotheses. One assumption that the projects share with Epstein is that the optimal times for such interventions may well be at the ages of onset of the Piagetian stages.

Cognitive Level Matching: Cognitive Demands

The concept of cognitive levels matching involves a complimentary concept of "the cognitive demands" of tasks. It is essential to ask what particular type of logical thinking or concepts are necessary to develop a new concept and thus come to understand the curricular task. For example, the child is asked what is the meaning of the simile "My shadow is like a piece of the night." The *cognitive demand* here requires ability to perform simple and multiple classifications. Mentally the child has to list the attributes of both shadows and night. Then the child has to search those lists to find out what shadows and nights have in common. This apparently simple task involves the child's ability to classify, to list attributes of objects, and to compare these lists and classifications.

While the ability to classify may be a logical prerequisite or necessary "demand" for this comprehension task, it is not sufficient in and of itself to insure the child's success. Children who lack the ability to classify, even if they can read the example, usually give literal answers. Typical answers include: "It means it is dark outside"; or "It's night time" or "Someone is chasing you down the street" (Arlin, 1978; Cometa & Eson, 1978). These literal responses are examples of "mismatches." The demands of the task are beyond the level of the students and so the students produce these answers.

Assessment

The Arlin Test of Formal Reasoning (1982) for cognitive levels involves the use of paper-and-pencil tests for concrete and formal reasoning (Arlin, 1982; Shayer, Adey & Wylan, 1981), and traditional clinical methods (Inhelder & Piaget, 1958, 1964). However, the emphasis in this article will be on the teacher's gradual development of strategies to do *informal* assessments of cognitive levels as evidence of these levels occurs in their daily interactions with students. For more information on the Formal Reasoning Test that includes prerequisites, 30 substates characteristics and curriculum example tasks, contact Dr. Arlin (reference note 5).

INFORMAL ASSESSMENTS

There are four general strategies which are derived from Piagetian and Neo-Piagetian research which provide the framework for these *informal* assessments. As the teacher develops a working knowledge of these research traditions, the strategies become the bridge between theory and practice. Both the knowledge base and the strategies gradually assist the teacher to acquire a *developmental perspective*. The knowledge base is acquired through opportunities provided teachers to come into contact with "powerful ideas" (Goodlad, 1983).

COGNITIVE LEVEL MATCHING:
A DEVELOPMENTAL PERSPECTIVE

A *developmental perspective* is a major component in the models of instruction (Arlin, reference note 1; Brooks, reference note 3). To have a developmental perspective is to consider curriculum and instruction in general, and the minute-by-minute interactions with children in particular from "the child's point-of-view" (Elkind, 1976). It was in these terms that Elkind described the contribution of child development to classroom practice:

> . . .one of the most important contributions child development can make is not so much particular contents, and principles of learning, as a general orientation towards children. What the developmentalist has to offer the teacher is first and foremost a *developmental perspective,* and techniques for exploring and revealing the child's own view of reality (1976, p. 53).

Hunt and Sullivan (1974) made a similar point when they suggested that for a developmental theory to be of help to teachers it "should specify the educational need of students at different stages of development and should distinguish between a child's immediate needs and his longterm requirements for growth" (p. 206). The same sentiment appears in earlier writings of Ausubel:

> . . .it is legitimate to evaluate the internal logic of instructional materials from the standpoint of their appropriateness for learners at a specific level of intellectual ability and of subject matter and developmental readiness (1968, p.29).

The strategies to be described below can be used at all levels of schooling. The initial focus and use of these strategies, however, was within middle schools. Students are typically eleven to fourteen years old in most middle school settings. Cognitive developmental researchers consistently report that approximately 50 percent of the adolescent and young adult population do not exhibit the use of formal operational thought when tested in the traditional clinical ways or in ways adapted by researchers (Keating, 1980; Maratono, 1977; Neimark, 1975, 1979).

It has often been suggested that the failure of adolescents to develop formal operational reasoning may be a function of the failure of educational institutions to provide appropriate impetus for such thought (Biggs & Collis, 1980; Kuhn, 1979). Despite this proposal, little systematic attempt has been made in public schools to adopt a developmental psychology of education and to structure school experiences to facilitate cognitive developmental change. The use of the following four strategies may be a first step toward the construction of an appropriate developmental curriculum that includes a *developmental perspective*.

Four General Strategies

The four general strategies are: (1) the identification of the child's "point-of-view"; (2) the analysis of children's responses in terms of the questions the children ask themselves; (3) the identification of specific Piagetian schemes, operations and concepts which comprise the "cognitive demands" of various Piagetian tasks; and (4) the analysis of children's faulty procedures or strategies. These general strategies are the first step in assisting teachers to reflect on the teaching act from a developmental perspective. They set up the possibility that out of that reflection might come action, adaptation of instruction and change.

First Strategy

The identification of the child's "point-of-view." It is by observing children, listening to children, and asking questions of children that opportunities are presented to observe tasks, experiences and concepts from their point-of-view. The emphasis of CLM on teachers acquiring a developmental perspective is focused directly on the teachers' coming in contact with the child's point-of-view. Unless tasks, concepts, one's own teaching are seen from this perspective, matching is an unattainable goal. Teachers, in planning lessons, attempt to anticipate children's responses, questions and difficulties with the lesson. Still, many lessons result in the unexpected. Children respond often in ways remarkably different from what adults expect. Piaget's clinical method takes this difference into account, expects it and uses it as a guide to children's thinking. Teachers use this method practically when they reflect on the child's point of view in their daily interactions. Three examples are drawn from three different age groups to illustrate this practical application of the clinical method.

An item on a Province-wide mathematics achievement test (Robitaille & Sherrill, 1977) taken by fourth graders at the beginning of the school year serves as our first example. The children were asked the question "Which group of dots is ½ shaded?" Approximately 60 percent of the children chose the correct answer where three dots were shaded and three were not. What was particularly interesting though was that the next most popular answer was the group of dots with two dots shaded and one dot unshaded. One possible explanation for the children's choice is that they related part-to-part rather than part to whole. They selected an answer of one and two rather than one-out-of-two. It is not uncommon in the Piagetian literature to report that approximately 40 percent of children age nine years are unable to coordinate part-whole relationships as represented in class inclusion problems and as possibly implied in this example.

The second example is taken from a seventh grade research study of children's comprehension of metaphors (Arlin, 1978). The young person is asked what is meant by the line "Tiptoe night comes down the lane, all alone, without a word, taking for his own again every little flower and bird." The student was an average student with no known learning disabilities and for whom English was his native language. The young man responded that it meant that "this man is walking down a path and he has a flower in his hand and a bird perched on his shoulder." Clearly he is giving a literal interpretation of a metaphoric expression.

Finally consider the eleventh grade honors physics course where students early in the year are asked to draw a curve which is a best fit for the data they generate in an experiment. A common response of students is to connect the dots rather than to draw a smooth curve using the dots as reference points (Stengel, reference note 4). The idea of "best fit" appears beyond the student who either considers her measurements to be exact or absolutely correct rather than subject to error. A second possible explanation for the student's graph may be that in most mathematics classes when students are asked to graph data from given equations, the graphs are always perfect if the calculations are correctly performed. The student always gets a perfect circle. Each of these three examples illustrates "point-of-view" at three different age levels.

Second Strategy

The analysis of children's responses in terms of the questions the children ask themselves. Papert is quoted as suggesting that children always correctly answer the questions they ask themselves (Sinclair & Kamii, 1970). This second strategy highlights the need for teachers and researchers to find out precisely the question that will guide a child or adolescent in the thinking process. Instead of focusing on a child's answer as "wrong" the strategy modelled for the teacher is to ask "What question is the child/adolescent asking herself for which this is the right answer?"

Consider, for example, the fourth grader who seemed to the teacher to know his basic multiplication facts and yet was stumped by the problem :" $2(4) + 4 = ?$" It turned out that he knew that 2 groups of 4 added to 4 were 12 but he couldn't understand why if this was the answer the problem hadn't been written "$3(4) = .$"

A second example is taken from a grade 6 class where a number of students insisted that 3/7's is larger than 3/6's because 7 is greater than 6. Possibly the question they were asking themselves was simply "which is the bigger number, 7 or 6?" rather than the question of which fraction represents the greater part of a whole.

Strauss (1981) reports an example of eighth grade students who were asked "if cold water and cold water are mixed together what will the resulting temperature be?" The students responded that cold water added to cold water gives cold water. The same students when later asked "what will the temperature of the mixture be when 10 degree water is added to 10 degree water?" They answered, "20 degrees" without hesitation. In this example the question that the students are asking themselves may well be "what is the sum of 10 + 10?" rather than "what is the temperature of the resulting mixture."

Third Strategy

The identification of specific Piagetian schemes, operations and concepts which comprise the "cognitive demands of various curriculum tasks." The teacher must first become acquainted with the definition of *class inclusion*. Basically class inclusion requires that the child be able to identify parts and a whole, and be able to coordinate part/whole relationships. Secondly, she learns how to clinically assess whether a child can do class inclusion tasks. Finally, she generates curriculum examples of tasks which have class inclusion as one of their cognitive demands; these might include "missing addend problems," finding the main idea in a paragraph, fractional concepts, states and their capitals.

Fourth Strategy

The analysis of children's faulty strategies or procedures. This strategy is similar to the second strategy. It differs in that it places emphasis on identifying the steps a child goes through in solving problems rather than simply on the child's questions.

The work of Case (1978) and other Neo-Piagetians emphasizes careful observations of children as they attempt to solve tasks. One then attempts to characterize their strategies, to compare these strategies with the strategies or procedures that an "expert" uses in solving a similar type of problem and then to compare the two as a clue to why the child is having difficulty with the problem. If a number of children are encouraged to describe aloud the steps they are going through as they attempt to solve problems, these sets of strategies can often be ordered from the least adequate to the most to assist the teacher in deciding what his instructional strategy will be. A fifth grade student who appeared to be having little difficulty with long division word problems was asked how he knew which number was the dividend and which number was the divisor. He replied that "the big number always goes inside and the little number always goes on the outside." While this was a strategy that served him well in fifth grade, he could begin to have problems once he begins division of decimals or fractions.

SUMMARY

Each of these four strategies represents an attempt to help teachers in their classrooms to come into contact with the child's point of view. A *developmental perspective* is simply that. CLM represents one way to bring this encounter about and to effect a fundamental change in teachers' view of teaching. If they can view instructional tasks from the child's point-of-view, the process of the match will have begun.

REFERENCE NOTES

1. Arlin, P. K. Symposium presentation at the Annual Meeting of the American Educational Research Association, Montreal, April, 1983.

2. Duckworth, E. Paper presented at the Annual Meeting of the American Educational Research Association, Montreal, April, 1983.

3. Brooks, M. Symposium presentation at the Annual Meeting of the American Educational Research Association, Montreal, April, 1983.

4. Stengel, P. Paper prepared as a course assignment, New York: Hofstra University, 1982.

5. For more information on the Arlin Test of Formal Reasoning, and the complete cognitive level matching system, contact Dr. Patricia Arlin, Department of Educational Psychology, The University of British Columbia, 2125 Main Mall, Vancouver, B.C. V6T 125, Canada.

REFERENCES

Arlin, P. K. *Metaphors and thought in children.* Vancouver, B.C.: Educational Research Institute of B.C., Research Report 78:1, 1978.

Arlin, P. K. A Multi-trait multi-method validity study of a test of formal reasoning. *Educational and Psychological Measurement*, 1983, *43*, 103-109.

Ausubel, D. P. *Educational psychology: a cognitive view.* New York: Holt, Rinehart, and Winston, 1968.

Biggs, J. B., & Collis, K. F. (Eds.). *Cognitive development and instruction.* New York: Academic Press, 1980.

Brooks, M., Fusco, E., & Grennon, J. Cognitive levels matching. *Educational Leadership*, 1983, *40*, 4-8.

Case, R. A developmentally based theory and technology of instruction. *Review of Educational Research*, 1978, *48*, 439-463.

Cometa, M., & Esom, M. Logical operations and metaphor interpretation: a Piagetian model. *Child Development*, 1978, 649-659.

Elkind, D. Egocentrism in adolescence. *Child Development*, 1969, *38*, 1025-1034.

Elkind, D. Child development in educational settings. *Educational Psychologist*, 1976, *12*, 49-58.

Epstein, H. T. Phrenoblysis: special brain and mind growth periods: I human brain and skill development. *Developmental Psychobiology*, 1974a, (u) 7, 207-216.

Epstein, H. T. Phrenoblysis: special brain and mind growth periods: II human mental development. *Developmental Psychobiology*, 1974b, *7*, 217-224.

Epstein, H. T. Growth spurts during brain development: implications for educational policy. In J. Chall (Ed.), *Education and the Brain*. Chicago: University of Chicago Press, 1978.

Epstein, H. T. Learning to learn: matching instruction to cognitive levels. *Principal*, 1981, *12*, 25-30.

Goodlad, J. I. A study of schooling: some implications for school improvement. *Phi Delta Kappan*, 1983, 552-560.

Hunt, D., & Sullivan, E. V. *Between Psychology and Education*. Hinsdale, Ill.: Dryden Press, 1974.

Inhelder, B., & Piaget, J. *The Growth of Logical Thinking from Childhood to Adolescence*. New York: Basic Books, 1958.

Inhelder, B., & Piaget, J. *The early growth of logic in the child: classification and seriation*. New York: Humanities Press, 1964.

Keating, D. Adolescent thinking. In J. Adelson (Ed.), *Handbook of Adolescence*. New York: John Wiley & Sons, 1980.

Kuhn, D. The significance of Piaget's formal operations stage in Education. *Journal of Education*, Boston University School of Education. 1979, *161*, 34-50.

Martorano, S. C. A developmental analysis of performance on Piaget's formal operations tasks. *Developmental Psychology*, 1977, *13*, 66-72.

Neimark, E. D. Intellectual development during adolescence. In F. D. Horowitz (Ed.), *Review of Child Development Research*, vol. 4. Chicago: University of Chicago Press, 1975.

Neimark, E. D. Current status of formal operations research. *Human Development*, 1979, *22*, 60-67. Robataille, D., &. Sherrill, J. *British Columbia Mathematics Assessment: A Summary*. Victoria, B.C.: Ministry of Education, 1977.

Shayer, M., & Wylam, H. The distribution of Piagetian stages of thinking in British middle and secondary school children: 14-16 year-old and sex differentials. *British Journal of Educational Psychology*. 1978, *48*, 62-70.

Sinclair, H., & Kamii, C. Implications of Piaget for the teaching of young children. *School Review.*, 1970, *78*, 62-70.

Strauss, S. Cognitive development in school and out. *Cognition*. 1981, *10*, 295-300.

Constructivism and Education:
The Child's Point-of-View

Martin Brooks, PhD
Esther Fusco, PhD

ABSTRACT. For several years, the Shoreham-Wading River school district has been involved in an in-service education program designed to sensitize teachers to the cognitive developmental theories of Piaget and to then apply these theories to classroom practices. The focus of the program has been "the child's point-of-view." Recognizing and understanding the child's point-of-view is seen as a critical element in helping teachers develop appropriate instructional programs for their pupils. This article describes ways in which educators have used their understandings of children's points of view in developing curriculum, structuring questions, interpreting test results and evaluating instruction.

SECTION I
COGNITIVE LEVEL MATCHING:
PHILOSOPHY AND IMPLEMENTATION

PHILOSOPHY

Although required reading in many graduate level educational methods courses, theories of Jean Piaget have rarely found their

Martin Brooks is Director of Elementary Education; Margaret Daugherty is an elementary special education teacher; Esther Fusco is a middle school reading teacher; Jacqueline Grennon is a middle school math/science teacher; Todd Kelley is an elementary music teacher and Bruce Lavalle is a middle school math/science teacher. All are staff members of the Shoreham-Wading River School District, Randall Road, Shoreham, NY 11786.

This article was coordinated and edited by the primary authors, Esther Fusco and Martin Brooks. Each section, however, was written by different Shoreham-Wading River staff members, and their names appear at the end of the sections they wrote. When names do not appear at the end of a section, it was written by Fusco and Brooks.

111

way into classroom practices. Indeed, theories of child development have traditionally been eschewed by people charged with both the development and implementation of curriculum, many of whom subscribe to the "more and quicker is better" school of thought. Consequently, much of our traditional curriculum is not well matched to the cognitive developmental abilities of the students from whom it is intended.

This dilemma forms the basis of the Cognitive Levels Matching (CLM) project in the Shoreham-Wading River (NY) school district. Participating teachers are exposed, through in-service education, to the theories of child development, with particular emphasis on constructivism—the notion that through direct, personal manipulation of objects and ideas, children construct knowledge. Similarly, teachers work together to construct for themselves ways in which the theories can be usefully translated to assist them in instruction. This approach is in contrast, to a large degree, with other notions which posit that individuals are best taught through methodologies which feed them a steady diet of facts and/or information.

The underlying hypothesis of the CLM project is that cognitive development can be facilitated by appropriate educational intervention, a proposition which admittedly makes some Piagetian theorists cringe. A central tenet of the project is matching. The appropriate educational intervention of which we speak is grounded in matching the cognitive demands of school experiences (including curriculum, questioning and testing) with the cognitive abilities of the students, while maintaining a degree of intellectual disequilibrium sufficient to keep the students motivated and challenged. The notion is similar to ideas espoused by Hunt (1961).

To achieve this match, teachers must (1) assess, in cognitive developmental terms, the cognitive demands of the curriculum, tests and questioning techniques they use, (2) assess the cognitive abilities of the students, and (3) attempt to match the two. It is important to note that we are not as interested in broad labels (concrete operational thinker, formal operational thinker, etc.) as we are in specific mental structures which students may or may not have yet developed (conservation of number, class inclusion, propositional reasoning, etc.). Piaget's stage theory, while interesting, does not appear to be as applicable to educational settings as are his descriptions of specific mental structures.

Critical to the assessment of the cognitive abilities of students is the teacher's capacity to recognize and understand the child's point-of-view. A teacher who asks a question designed to elicit one "correct" answer tells children, either directly or subtly, that they are "right" or "wrong." Children who are "right" are reinforced; children who are "wrong" are frustrated and/or disappointed. Teachers who seek to understand the child's point of view, however, give more value, both directly and subtly, to the answers of all children by pursuing the child's line of reasoning through additional questions which require the child to elaborate on and explain his/her answers. For example, if a child who answers "3" to the question "How much is $2 + 2$?" is told that he/she is wrong, and that the answer is actually "4," not much learning occurs. However, if the teacher mediates the situation by asking the child to explain how the answer "3" was reached, the child is given more of an opportunity to rethink the problem. If still unable to reach the answer "4" through mental processes, the teacher may suggest the child test the answer again with blocks, chain links or unifix cubes. Upon re-solving the problem through direct manipulation of objects, the child is more likely to answer "4." In addition, the process of solving the problem over again in a directly verifiable manner will enable the child to construct new knowledge which can then be applied to future problems requiring similar solutions. Without valuing the child's point of view, the teacher loses this opportunity for the child to construct new knowledge. It is for this reason that we have selected as the main theme of this article "the child's point-of-view."

The remainder of this article will be structured with "the child's point-of-view" as its common thread. Following a brief description of the project, Section II (Fusco and Lavalle) will discuss the child's point-of-view vis-à-vis the process of curriculum adaptation. Section III (Grennon and Kelley) will discuss the role of inquiry in discovering the child's point-of-view. Section IV (Daugherty) will describe the role of testing in understanding the child's point-of-view. Section V (Brooks) will discuss how an understanding of the child's point-of-view changes traditional administrative practices, particularly the process of teacher evaluation.

IMPLEMENTATION

For the past three years, our district has been involved in a voluntary, in-service education program designed to sensitize teachers to the process of cognitive development. The project was initiated by staff members who attended a summer graduate course conducted respectively by Patricia Arlin of the University of British Columbia and Herman Epstein of Brandeis University. The course was devoted to the relationship between Piaget's theory of child development and recent research related to the human brain. Approximately 135 of a possible 215 district staff members have currently participated in the Cognitive Levels Matching Project. As stated above, the in-service education program in our district is designed to teach teachers to (1) determine the cognitive demands of school-based curricula, (2) assess the cognitive abilities of students, and (3) attempt to match the two. It is important to reiterate here that the purpose of the program is not to create an environment which limits teachers' perceptions of students' cognitive abilities. Rather, the process encourages teachers to generate, for their students, an enhancing degree of intellectual disequilibrium. This approach reduces the frustrations which often accompany teacher/student interactions and provides intellectual challenges which allow students to actively seek the construction of knowledge.

CLM is based on Piaget's constructivist theory of its application to educational settings by teachers who are learning to understand the ways children think. Inhelder and Piaget (1969) state:

> In the development of the child, there is no preestablished plan, but a gradual evolution in which each innovation is dependent upon the previous one. Adult thought might seem to provide a preestablished model, but the child does not understand adult thought until he has reconstructed it, and thought is itself the result of an evolution carried on by several generations, each of which has gone through childhood. (p.157)

IN-SERVICE EDUCATION

The literature on teacher change was consulted in order to establish a program which would encompass a sound theoretical foundation for our instruction. Thus, the in-service courses are structured into three levels. The first level, a six-credit graduate course, concentrates on Piagetian theory and its relationship to the curriculum and the child's development of reasoning abilities. The second-level is a follow-up course designed to examine and elaborate, in detail, the principles of the initial course. Finally, an advanced level course is offered to encourage teachers to explore the cognitive demands of specific curriculum areas while systematically evaluating their own teaching performances when presenting the material. Teachers are paid a stipend for their participation in all three courses, and are encouraged to form partnerships to generate feedback on their implementation of the techniques to the classroom.

We hypothesize that the training will enable teachers to facilitate the cognitive development of their students through more appropriate educational intervention. Thus, by the conclusion of the courses, participants are expected to:

1. Identify the mental structures associated with each of the four stages in Piaget's model of cognitive development.
2. Critique Piaget's stage model with respect to general educational implications.
3. Analyze student's work for information relevant to cognitive levels.
4. Examine curriculum and their own teaching and questioning styles in terms of assumed and implied cognitive demands.
5. Generate examples of the specific cognitive schemes identified in the Piagetian model through their own teaching and content areas.

The objectives of the courses are accomplished in the give and take of a regular, diverse classroom. CLM is neither the sum of curricular units adapted nor the degree of homogeneity one can impose on a class. Rather, it is the teacher's ability to perceive, think and act spontaneously in a classroom situation while employing the developmental principles of the training.

SECTION II
THE CHILD'S POINT-OF-VIEW:
CURRICULAR ADAPTATION

As mentioned in the preceding article by Arlin, a *developmental perspective* which seeks to understand the child's point-of-view, provides (1) a framework for cognitively analyzing curriculum, (2) data about the cognitive abilities of students, and (3) a mechanism for developing more appropriate methodological strategies for instruction. Such a perspective we have discovered, reduces teacher and student frustration.

Teachers often experience frustration when students are unable to grasp the concepts they are expected to easily understand. As a result, teachers often find themselves exhausted and disappointed even though they have presented comprehensive and detailed explanations. Why don't students understand? We feel that students often struggle with concepts that are inappropriate for their level of cognitive development. Consequently, they are unable to grasp the meaning of many concepts beyond a superficial level and do not internalize the information so that it can be applied at a later date.

Piaget's developmental theories have presented us the opportunity to transform, to some extent, this situation. Inhelder and Piaget (1964) write:

> The principal goal of education is to create men who are capable of doing new things, not simply of repeating what other generations have done—men who are creative, inventive, and discoverers. The second goal of education is to form minds which can be critical, can verify, and not accept everything they are offered. The great danger today is of slogans, collective opinions, ready-made trends of thought. We have to be able to resist individually, to criticize, to distinguish between what is proven and what is not. So we need pupils who are active, who learn early to find out by themselves, partly by their own spontaneous activity and partly through materials we set up for them; who learn early to tell what is verifiable and what is simply the first idea to come to them. (p. 5)

Through the training, the teachers create methodologies which enables them to present cognitively appropriate tasks. Such tasks allow students to enhance their repertories of experiences, and organize and integrate new learning into their own cognitive structures. In the curriculum areas of science, math and language arts, natural opportunities occur. Providing a diversity of questions is helpful since students in any class will range in cognitive abilities. Appropriately matched questions allow students to show what they do and do not understand, and reduce their anxiety about learning. It is important to note that all responses are valued by the instructor since they represent the students' thinking at the moment, and facilitate the teachers' modification of future curriculum. Once the matching and listening occur with regularity, students are more easily able to attend to responses that are not consistent with their own thinking. The atmosphere in classrooms becomes more dynamic and cooperative because of the increased sharing and greater appreciation of everyone's contributions. Specific curriculum examples are presented to illustrate this point.

EXAMPLE 1

The book *Sounder* by William Armstrong (1969) is often used in upper elementary, middle, and junior high schools. Students often experience difficulty comprehending this book. *Sounder* tells the story of a poor black sharecropper's family living in the South during the Depression. The father steals a ham to feed his starving family. He is caught by the sheriff and his men who beat and insult him in front of the family. The dog, Sounder, tries to protect the father and is shot by the sheriff. Somehow the dog and the family survive. In order to comprehend the essence of this story, the students must have the ability to do some high level thinking. They must go beyond the details, or literal level, and do correlational reasoning, coordinate two or more frames of reference simultaneously and think propositionally. Some students are able to reason thusly, while others are not. The experience of all students, regardless of ability, is enhanced when a range of questions is presented. This range is important because it allows (1) students to be involved in an analytical process and (2) the teacher to listen to students' responses and cognitively evaluate them in order to plan for the students' future interactions. The following are three excerpts from a discussion on *Sounder:*

(1)

Teacher: Why does the mother sing this song? "You've gotta walk that lonesome valley. You've gotta walk it by yourself. Ain't nobody else gonna walk for you. . ."
Matt: It was pretty lonesome back then. He had nothing to do.

(2)

Teacher: Why do you think no one has a name in the story except Sounder?
Matt: That was what the whole book was about. The story is about Sounder.

(3)

Teacher: Imagine the dangers the boy faces on the road when he goes looking for his father. How does he justify his search to his mother? Why does the mother allow him to go?
Matt: He was always afraid to see other people.
Teacher: To see people?
Matt: On the street he's afraid of them and now he won't be.

Based on Matt's responses, and recognition of his point of view, the teacher was able to infer that he would be helped by curriculum experiences which focused on detail and selected as the vehicle for this focus the concept of characterization. Thus, future reading activities contained material which assisted him in thinking about the multi-dimensional attributes of a character. Further, the teacher worked on synchronizing the character in a story to the events and issues which were shared. A record sheet structured in the following manner was used.

Name of Character	Qualities or Attributes of the Character	Event or Scene

EXAMPLE 2

In addition to appropriate questions, students need the opportunity to work with content and materials in a hands-on fashion. Currently in math and science, students are provided time to work with carefully selected materials which present specific notions and which enable them to build their own theories related to the topic. They are encouraged to pose questions which can be answered through experimentation with materials. They note and respond to their physical properties and their non-physical characteristics. This type of sequential reinforcement also expands students' repertories of experiences. They are able to relate back to previous experiences in other units and link them to new units, and oftentimes they are able to project ahead to future cases. A goal of this hands-on, sequential process is to enable students to listen to and understand their peers' reactions to experiments. Often, these reactions assist students in expanding their own viewpoints.

For example, in a culminating Solar Energy Unit, students performed demonstrations and experiments which were arranged to reinforce and verify scientific concepts that had been presented throughout the year. A final project was outlined which allowed students to apply the principles discussed. The application required students to build an energy-efficient, three dimensional model home. The expectations for each student were dependent upon their cognitive abilities as displayed through on-going class activities. Thus, the houses varied from very simple but efficient to highly technical designs.

The solar energy homes allowed students to tangibly test, apply, and verify their points of view. It presented the opportunity for meaningful learning since students were intensely involved with recalling, recreating, and constructing knowledge during the process. Students discussed and defended their notions about efficient solar homes. They presented their completed projects with pride and certainty. Their presentations assisted the teacher in evaluating their cognitive growth during the year. Below are two homes designed and constructed by students (Figure 1 and 2).

EXAMPLE 3

Eighth grade students participated in a letter writing unit in which each student received the name of an elderly person who lived in an adult home. The students were asked to write and visit the adult once every few weeks. The adults were selected because they had not had a visitor in over a year and did not often receive mail.

The goals of the project were to develop the student's (1) ability

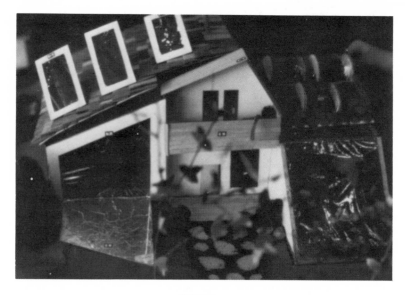

FIGURE 1

to write letters, (2) sense of audience, (3) feeling of usefulness by attending to the needs of others, (4) sense of responsibility, and (5) relationship with elderly people.

In observing, listening to, and reading students' writing, the teacher learned a great deal about the students' points of view. For example, several students were surprised to see their cards or letters displayed in the elderly persons' rooms. One student said: "You know Edith has the card I made in school in her room." A discussion ensued about what he imagined would happen to his card once he put the addressed envelope in the school's outgoing mail box. Later, this student responded to three newspaper ads and received information from each company.

Some students independently began to prepare special activities for their adults. As they discovered the adults' interests, some students immediately began to pursue them and then planned future activities accordingly. Finally, one student commented: "Teenagers and old people are alike. We have no real jobs that make a difference. Our society doesn't really need either of us." As a result of this comment, poetry writing sessions were set up so that this student could pursue her feelings about the correlation between age and treatment by society.

After each visit to the adult home, students shared their experiences. The sharing was a significant component of the process, which assisted students in developing awareness of other viewpoints about the elderly. Some students were able to take another's frame of reference (their adult), and empathetically justify their opinions. It further permitted them to elaborate upon and evaluate diverse situations (social security, death, aging, hospitalization). The sharing assisted the teacher in determining which cognitive structures needed support.

Esther Fusco
Bruce Lavalle

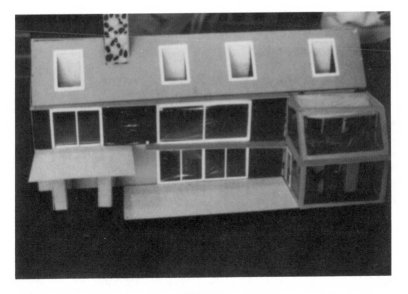

FIGURE 2

SECTION III
THE CHILD'S POINT-OF-VIEW: QUESTIONING

VIGNETTE

Teacher: How are trains and cars the same?

Alison: Well, they both have steering wheels.

Teacher: What do you mean by that?

Alison: You know. It's the round thing in a car that you turn to make it go.

Teacher: Well, I'll tell you the truth. I've never been in a train engine before, but someone told me that there are no steering wheels on trains.

Mark: My grandfather took me into the engine of a train once and I didn't see a steering wheel.

Brian: But, I was on a train.

Teacher: Tell us what you saw.

Brian: Well, I was only in the sitting part. But I thought I saw into the driver part and I saw a steering wheel.

Teacher: Now, I am going to ask you to predict. Do you think the driver could steer the train to our school and pick us up?

Angela: No, there are no tracks here.

Teacher: Who agrees with Angela?

After a discussion in which many opinions were elicited regarding the purpose and function of tracks, the teacher decided to conduct an experiment whereby he took a toy train and rolled it down an incline: First without tracks, and then with curved tracks. Demonstrating in front of the children, the teacher released the train which followed a random path without the tracks and a fixed path with the tracks. The teacher then asked: "When did the train turn?" Most children responded: "When the train was on the tracks." The teacher reposed the initial question: "Do you think trains need steering wheels to turn?" The child, Mark, maintained his original opinion; two other children in the class who originally said "yes" changed their minds: all the remaining children still said yes. The teacher, modeling a still perplexed orientation, suggested a field trip to the local train station so that the children could look into the engine and discover for themselves whether trains have steering wheels.

OVERVIEW

This vignette describes an instance in which, through probing questioning, a teacher sought to discover the points of view of the children in his class. The teacher's discovery that children disagreed as to the existence of steering wheels on trains presented the teacher with an impromptu opportunity to set up a structure within which the children could critically consider some disequilibrating ideas. Through the experiment with tracks, two students reasoned that the tracks determined the pathway of the train and stated that steering wheels are not present. The other students were not swayed by the results of the experiment. By the arrangement of the field trip, all children were given the opportunity to experience first hand the object of their curiosity.

The role of questioning holds a fundamental position in the classroom. There exists a critical relationship between teacher inquiry and the child's affective and cognitive development. In terms of affective development, the method of question asking is laden with meaning: a teacher who can share his sense of excitement about discovery establishes the importance of questioning as a valued classroom endeavor. The child perceives the teacher as an inquiring individual who seeks understanding. Conversely, the nature of the teacher's responses when *children* pose questions holds the awesome power of either energizing the inquisitive nature of the child or squelching that natural proclivity. In terms of cognitive development, not only does the nature of the teacher-directed questions influence the child's predisposition to learn, but it provides an environment that promotes thinking (Sigel, 1979).

How can the environment promote intellectual growth? *Does* the environment promote intellectual growth? Although environmental factors contribute significantly to the development of both cognition and affect within the child (Zimmerman, 1981), we stress that it is the child's active *engagement* with a mediated environment which furthers the child's development. The teacher provides this mediation through selection and presentation of materials, the scheduling of options, the provision of various levels of reading materials, and, most central to this section of the paper, questioning techniques. Questioning techniques are most helpful when they are used to engage the child in discourse which is reflective of the child's point of view. A goal of the teacher is to understand the information rendered by the child through discussion in terms of the child's perspective. This dynamic process of teacher/child interaction is ongoing and requires teacher sensitivity. This sensitivity is based on the teacher's ability to synthesize the underlying psychology of the child with the demands of the classroom. Thus, understanding the child's point of view has two functions: (1) a broad understanding of the typical characteristics of children's perspectives at various ages guides the teacher in the selection of appropriate curricula; and (2) at a child specific level, the teacher's quest to understand the child's point of view guides the formulation of initial and follow-up questions.

THE CHILD'S POINT-OF-VIEW

Our model, rooted in the theories and observations of Inhelder and Piaget (1964), attempts to track the development of the child's point-of-view. As children enter school they typically demonstrate an egocentric view. Limited in their ability to take another's viewpoint, they often judge situations from their own perspective while disregarding the perspective of others. During the elementary school grades children's ability to respond to the needs of another gradually increases. Oftentimes, the abilities of children in the middle and high schools are expanded to include hypothetical thinking and divergent lines of argument. Therefore, this process gradually shifts the child's personal point of view to a social one in which the individual reconciles her individuality with societal and cultural expectations. Cognizant of these broad characteristics, the teacher constantly modifies and adapts curricula, most particularly curricular questions that enable him to understand the child's point-of-view.

TEACHER INTERVENTION

What is this questioning process? (1) The teacher uses *elaboration techniques*. The teacher in the vignette asked, "What do you mean by that," "Tell us what you saw." He avoided closeout statements such as "No, that's not the answer I'm looking for." In order to spark the child's motivation to elaborate, he posed contradictions. (2) The teacher uses *cognitive terminology*. The teacher in the vignette asked the children to predict, and he incorporated the word into the question. (3) The teacher *shifts the presentation of the lesson, as well as criteria for student evaluation, to use methodologies and strategies relative to the children's responses.* The teacher in the vignette, realizing that the experiment in conjunction with his question regarding steering wheels required reasoning beyond the abilities of his students, suggested a field trip for visual verification. For 5-year-old children, "hypothesis testing" through visual verification is more likely within their grasp than the isolation of variables necessary for understanding the experiment as it relates to whether or not trains have steering wheels. (4) The teacher *encourages children's questions and children/children interaction.* The teacher in the vignette asked the children to respond to each other's statements: "Who agrees with Angela?" is an example. (5) The teacher *is sensitive to the knowledge/experiential frameworks that the children bring to the curricular task.* The teacher in the vignette respectfully acknowledged the children's beliefs and prior experiences with trains. Based on the information the teacher received, he made plans to expand their background in ways appropriate to their age and cognitive level. Through the use of these techniques, the teacher gains some degree of access to the child's frame of reference.

There are many paradigms and models which present questioning taxonomies, the most commonly used probably being Bloom's Taxonomy of Educational Objectives (1956). While some educational models have viewed these categories as synchronous with developmental stages, we hold that these categories occur throughout each developmental stage. School age children, at all stages, recall information, translate symbols into meaning, interpret, apply knowledge to problems, and are capable of the "higher order" functions of analyzing data, synthesizing ideas and evaluating decisions. For example, first grade children in most classrooms are assigned jobs in order to understand the role of work in a social setting. The following example describes Dennis, whose job it is to sponge off all the table tops and who fulfills his responsibilities vigorously. After a long uphill walk on a fieldtrip, Dennis proclaimed with a spark of insight, "Today, my *legs* are doing all the work."

How did Dennis' epiphany occur? The teacher, in attempting to enable Dennis to discover similarities between different types of work, mediated the situation by stating, "Wow, this hill is steeper than I thought. We did a lot of work." This statement prompted Dennis' response, which helped the teacher to realize that Dennis was capable of analyzing the differences and similarities between these two seemingly disparate activities. Similarly, but considering many more variables, a high school biology student analyzes the comparative functions of body systems in various species, or a middle school English student analyzes character development in terms of, for example, emotional entanglement.

SUMMARY

We posit that the teacher's *developmental perspectives* can be used productively to build firm bases upon which children's intellectual potentials are enhanced. In order to challenge the full range of intellect, we must structure situations that capitalize on the child's developmental abilities. Our goal is to integrate cognitive developmental perspectives into a rigorous educational setting: rigorous meaning one which incorporates reasoning demands such as delineated by Sigel's Distancing Questioning Strategies (1979).

Achieving this goal is dependent upon two steps. First, one must create an educational milieu which promotes interactions between children and children, children and teacher, and children and materials. Understanding the child's point-of-view is a fundamental precursor to this step. Second, and most significantly, the teacher's questioning of the child must enable the child to recognize contradictions, identify relationships, formulate hypotheses and conceptualize ways of solving problems. Such activities promote the development of cognition.

Jackie Grennon
Todd Kelley

SECTION IV
THE CHILD'S POINT-OF-VIEW: TESTING

This section will focus on the effect CLM has had on the perspective and processes of an elementary school's Child Study Team (CST). This team is a multi-disciplinary, diagnostic/prescriptive group which meets weekly to discuss, evaluate, and adapt the instructional programs for children who appear to be having difficulties in standard classroom situations. When a child is perceived by a teacher or parent as having difficulty in the academic or social aspects of a classroom, a referral is made. The CST is composed of the school psychologist, special education teacher, speech/language therapist, reading specialist, nurse, the referring classroom teacher and the building principal. Input is also available from special area teachers, such as the music and physical education teachers. In an effort to assess a child's strengths and weaknesses, the team discusses the teacher's perceptions, the child's standardized test scores, social skills and maturation. The intent, at this point, is to see if and where there is difficulty and to specify the nature of the problem via comprehensive psychoeducational testing, physical examinations, and continued observations and monitoring. Approximately one month after this initial meeting, the parents are invited to a follow-up meeting at which time evaluations and impressions are discussed and adaptations in the child's program are recommended.

What has been described above is a standard procedure that has been in practice in our district for a number of years. It predated the CLM project in the district. What has changed since the initiation of the project is the effort by team members to gather and attempt to apply information regarding the child's thought processes from a common developmental perspective, that of Piaget. Traditionally, the team questioned whether the "problems" identified by a standard psychoeducational battery were related to physical, linguistic, academic, processing or emotional difficulties. Now, the team also questions if the child is ready for the tasks being presented, in a cognitive developmental sense. A common developmental perspective, combined with data derived from a psychoeducational evaluation, focuses discussions on the child's abilities and points of view. While testing, a child's cognitive abilities are assessed not only through a standard Piagetian interview, but also through careful focus on responses to questions posed through an inquiry method. Standardized evaluation devices tend to militate against divergent answers. In fact, they tend to militate against most answers, except the "correct" few required during test normalization. Tests, in general, do not appear to focus on the child's points-of-view, but rather seek the answers given most often by the normalization sample. By questioning a child to determine his/her point of view, one is able to assess the thinking behind the response. Child Study Team members question a child's response on test items and actively listen for the "why" of the child's reasoning processes and not just for a particular answer. CST members make use of the fundamental conflict between test construction and the child's view of the situation. While adhering to the standardized protocols and scoring procedures, team members sensitively probe responses to see "why," "how," and "what if." For example, why did a child respond in a particular way to a "fund of information" question on an intelligence test? How did the examiner attempt to see the possible incongruence between the question asked and the question the child actually heard?

Another change in the CST process is the inclusion of a standard Piagetian interview. The basic concrete operational tasks of conversation, classification, and seriation are presented to our elementary population and the child's reasoning is explored in order to tap the child's point-of-view. The CST then meets with the parents to report the findings and impressions. A more holistic discussion of the child occurs, with standard test scores, of course, considered and weighed, but also with the benefit of insights about the child's reasoning filtered through a common developmental framework. This information is the basis for planning an educational program which is rich in opportunities and will enhance cognitive and affective development.

Margaret Daugherty

SECTION V
THE CHILD'S POINT-OF-VIEW: ADMINISTRATION

During the last several years, much has been written about effective schools, and about the role of the principal in contributing to effectiveness. One criterion for effectiveness consistently identified in the literature has to do with instructional leadership. Schools in which principals are actively involved in defining, developing and implementing the instructional components of their schools' programs are generally considered more effective than schools in which the principals view themselves primarily as managers.

The traditional model of administration and supervision involves the principal in the teaching process on two levels: staff-wide and teacher-specific. Staff-wide responsibilities typically include goal setting, curriculum development and evaluation of programs. Teacher-specific activities generally include goal setting meetings, observations, follow-up conferences and end-of-year evaluation meetings.

This traditional model of administration and supervision generates little collaboration between teacher and principal because the focus of the process is that largely subjective, nebulous factor referred to as "quality" of teaching. The process is threatening for teachers because their behaviors and actions are scrutinized and criticized. Meetings between principals and teachers are often marked by defensiveness on the part of teachers ("You are not aware of what preceded the lesson you observed"), and superficiality on the part of principals ("Your bulletin boards aren't current and the aim of your lesson wasn't written on the board").

The developmental perspective taught through the Cognitive Levels Matching project offers principals an opportunity to assume broader responsibilities: it enables principals to become involved in learning as well as teaching. The model of administration and supervision fostered by a CLM perspective alters teacher/principal interactions in constructive and productive ways. Principals are trained to focus on both teaching *and* learning, and the delicate interplay between them. This perspective encourages the principal to examine two viewpoints; the point of view of the teacher *and* the point-of-view of the child.

Like the traditional model, administration and supervision with a CLM perspective also involves the principal on two levels: staff-wide and teacher-specific. However, the nuances of principal involvement are changed significantly. Staff-wide responsibilities of the principal include development and articulation of a philosophical shift in emphasis from curriculum development to curriculum analysis. Teachers and principals jointly analyze school curricula from the child's point-of-view; e.g., are materials developmentally appropriate for the students with whom they are used? Teacher-specific activities include conferences and meetings similar to those described under the traditional model. Again, however, the nuances are changed. When the principal observes a class, the child's point-of-view becomes a central theme. This means that the principal looks at both student response and teacher behavior as factors contributing to the dynamic teaching/learning process, and is more sensitive to and respectful of the role of student cognitive abilities in this process.

For example, under the traditional model of administration and supervision, the principal focuses solely or primarily on teacher behaviors and classroom materials. If the behaviors and materials are deemed appropriate, students who do not "get" the point of the lesson are frequently perceived as inadequate.

Principals with a CLM perspective, however, are taught to be more sensitive to the process of cognitive development. Rather than inadequate, students are viewed as not being cognitively ready for certain materials and/or concepts. This perspective forms the basis for ensuing teacher/principal interactions about lessons observed. The focus of these interactions becomes children, and the various points of view they demonstrate on a daily basis. Teachers are less threatened because (1) they are not the sole objects of administrative observations, (2) they are encouraged to emphasize in their discussions with administrators that which they know best—their students, and (3) both the teacher and principal are collaboratively working toward the same goal: understanding and assisting the learning of each student.

Through this process, teachers and principals have a common base of knowledge, share a common perspective and speak a common language about children. For example, stating that a particular question required the responder to be capable of propositional reasoning and was therefore too demanding is less threatening to the teacher and more productive for the student than stating that the responder seemed disinterested and uninvolved in the lesson.

Principal sensitivity to children's points of view, then, enables collaboration with teachers in effecting a better match between the cognitive demands of curriculum and the cognitive abilities of students.

Martin Brooks

SECTION VI
CONCLUSION

It is said that Piaget's interest in cognitive development was initiated while he was working with Binet on norming an intelligence test. He noticed that on certain questions disproportionate percentages of children were choosing the same "incorrect" response. Upon further study and reflection, Piaget reasoned that these "incorrect" responses actually indicated the thinking patterns typical of most children of a particular chronological age. He concluded that the children were not "incorrect," but were instead demonstrating the prevailing point of view for children of a particular stage of development. For them, then, the "incorrect" answer was in fact "correct" for the manner in which the children interpreted the question they posed themselves.

Whether one accepts or disagrees with Piaget's theories, one must recognize, as a significant contribution, his valuing the points of view of children. This perspective, which is lacking in traditional educational settings, creates new opportunities for improving instruction and, we think, facilitating cognitive development. Teachers, who are sensitive to the mental processes demonstrated by their students, are able to cognitively challenge students with appropriate experiences. Children display for us their points of view on a daily basis. Our challenge, as educators, is to recognize that which is displayed and structure opportunities for them to construct new knowledge.

REFERENCES

Armstrong, W. *Sounder*. New York: Harper & Row, Publishers, 1969.
Bloom, B.S. *Taxonomy of Educational Objectives: The Classification of Educational Goals. Handbook 1 Cognitive Domain*. New York: McKay, 1956.

Hunt, J. *Intelligence and Experience*. New York: Ronald Press, 1961.

Inhelder, B. & Piaget, J. *The Growth of Logical Thinking From Childhood to Adolescence*. New York: Humanities Press, 1964.

Inhelder, B. & Piaget, J. *The Psychology of the Child*. New York: Basic Books, Inc., 1969.

Piaget, J. Development and Learning. In R. Ripple & A. Rockcastle (Eds.), *Piaget Rediscovered*, Ithaca, New York: Cornell University Press, 1964.

Sigel, I.E., & Saunders, R. An Inquiry Into Inquiry: Question Asking as An Instructional Model. In L.G. Katz (Ed.), *Current Topics in Early Childhood Education* (Vol. 2). Norwood, New Jersey: Ablex Publishing Corp., 1979.

Zimmerman, B. Social Learning Theory and Cognitive Construction. In I. Sigel, D. Brodzinsk, & R. Golinkoff (Eds.), *New Directions In Piagetian Theory And Practice*. Hillsdale, New Jersey: Lawrence Erlbaum Associates, Publishers, 1981.

The Relationship Between Language Development and Brain Development

Christine C. Pappas, PhD

ABSTRACT. The relationship between language development and brain development is examined. First, major characteristics of contemporary views on oral and written language development are presented. The the predominant ways in which language function and the brain have been investigated are critically reviewed. This review covers morphological findings, the commissurotomy studies, dichotic listening and visual half-field studies, EEG and cerebral blood flow studies, as well as topics on the development of lateralization and brain growth. The last section concludes that very little information exists about the relationship between language development and brain development, and argues that implications for education which invoke findings from recent brain research should be approached with great caution.

The task set forth by the title is a formidable one—many books and articles have focused on the topic of language development, on the topic of brain development, and even on the topic of the relationship between the two. At best, all that can be done here, then, is to provide a sketchy, but hopefully enough of an accurate view, of the contemporary stance on the relationship between language development and brain development.

Many of the issues having to do with the relationship between developing human language capabilities and the organization or structure of the brain—issues of the evolution of the mind, lateralization of function, plasticity of the brain and recovery of function, to mention a few—are complex and even controversial; *conclusive* answers about the relationship of language function and brain structure are not as yet forthcoming. Too frequently, simplistic ac-

Christine C. Pappas, Assistant Professor, University of Oregon, Division of Teacher Education, Eugene, OR 97403.

133

counts have led to spurious and misleading conclusions about brain function. Consequently, a major goal of the following review of recent findings and theoretical speculations about language and brain development will be to include various caveats whose purpose will be to acknowledge and remind us of the complexity and unsettled state of affairs.

The chapter will be organized into three major sections. The first section will present the major characteristics of contemporary views on language development. Both oral and written language will be covered but the predominant focus will be on oral language development. The second section will consist of a critical review of recent theoretical and research findings on brain research and an attempt to summarize the major conclusions concerning the relationship between language development and brain development. The final section will suggest clinical and/or educational implications based on these conclusions.

CONTEMPORARY VIEWS ON LANGUAGE DEVELOPMENT

A Brief History on Language Development

Attempts to explain language development are always tied to underlying assumptions about the nature of language itself and about the particular way in which it should be studied. A brief history of the research on language development, therefore, can provide a useful initial guide to current views on language development.

Historically, an early emphasis in the research of child language was one of describing the *form* of language. To a great extent, Chomsky's early work (1959, 1965) arguing against the prevailing psychological association learning theory to account for language acquisition was responsible for this emphasis. During this era, a host of studies concentrated upon documenting children's acquisition of all kinds of forms from negatives and interrogateries (Bellugi, 1967; Bellugi-Klimo, 1968) to grammatical morphemes (Berko, 1958) to certain aspects of syntax—those which are exceptions of the minimal distance principle (C. Chomsky, 1969)—as some examples.

Following this form emphasis, studies began to include an investigation into the child's learning of the *content* of language. Indeed, it became apparent that understanding children's acquisition of grammatical knowledge would require an attention to the *meanings* children expressed. For example, Bloom (1970) noted that the same form, *mommy sock,* uttered by Kathryn in Stage I represented two different semantic-syntactic categories: possessor-possessed ("Kathryn picked up her mother's sock") and agent-object ("Mother was putting Kathryn's sock on Kathryn"). Thus, investigators, influenced by generative semantic theorists such as Fillmore (1968) and Chafe (1970), began to include semantic explanations for early child multi-word language (Brown, 1973) as well as one-word utterances (Greenfield & Smith, 1976) in the child's developing grammatical knowledge. In addition, studies investigating children's acquisition of extensional word meanings (Clark, 1973; Nelson, 1973; Rosch, 1973) flourished during this time.

Unlike the focus on form which tends to emphasize only *linguistic* details of the internal organization of a formal system, the focus on semantics tended to move outward towards a consideration of the relationships between language and other activities such as thinking about, and referring to, objects and events in the world around us (Wells, 1981). Thus, during this semantic era two major things occurred. First, many investigators (Brown, 1973; Bloom, 1970; Bloom, Lightbown, & Hood, 1975; Nelson, 1973) began to rely on Piaget's sensorimotor intelligence to provide the cognitive foundation for early word meanings and sentence constructions of young children. Secondly, beginning with Bloom's study (1970), semantic *intentions,* attributed to the child's utterances on the basis of clues and behavior found in the context of situation, became a focus of research.

Then in the 1970s, another switch in emphasis occurred. How children learn to *use* language began to be explored. Up until then much of the work in child language relied upon two kinds of assumptions: (1) that adult contribution into the child's language learning process was fairly insignificant; and (2) that socially appropriate use of language emerged later in the child's development. The first assumption stemmed from Chomsky's notion about the language acquisition device (the LAD). That is, inherent in his ideas about the innate nature of the LAD was the implication that the child needed only a language environment consisting of any random adult utterances for language to be acquired. The second assumption originated from Piaget's (1926) characterization of young children's language as being egocentric. The latest research focus, then, explored children's *use* of language and began to question both of these sorts of assumptions. Such a focus included investigating specifically the nature of the mother's language *to* the child (Snow, 1972), for example, and examining the interactions between the adult and child in order to document the developing discourse abilities of children—i.e., their ability to obtain information from a prior linguistic message and then form a contingent message (Bloom, Rocissano, & Hood, 1976). Moreover, new considerations about language functions in social situations indicated that the requisite communicative foundation for the development of language began at the very beginning of a child's life: joint attention and action between the mother and the child is the ontogenesis of speech acts (Bruner, 1975a; Dore, 1974) and learning to mean (Halliday, 1975).

While most investigators in the language development field today acknowledge that the work done on transformational-generative (Chomsky, 1959, 1965) grammar has increased our understanding of the internal organization of the language system, they believe that this abstract knowledge of linguistic form has prevented us from finding out about the ways in which people actually communicate through language and about the relationship between linguistic messages and the context in which they occur. Thus, the development of *linguistic competence* as an area of concern has waned and has been replaced by an interest in the development of *communicative competence*—how children learn to use language for different purposes in different contexts. Certain notions—"innateness," "intentions," "prespeech cognition"—have been incorporated into the contemporary emphasis on the social uses of language, but not necessarily the same way. To understand how they are now conceived of requires that we examine in more detail that research which has focused on *prelinguistic* development.

Prelinguistic Communication

What is the role or significance of the child's pre-speech communication system? Whatever the theoretical bias—innate or empiricist—any explanation of language development in general must somehow deal with this question (Bruner, 1975a, 1975b). What is the nature of this system and what aspects of it will provide the continuity from pre-speech to language?

The need to better understand these preconditions for languages has led to a series of studies of the behavior of infants and neonates. The findings of these studies indicate that babies appear to be innately endowed with two kinds of abilities. The infant, first of all, is inherently capable of differentiating himself from the world. By their reaching and orienting behaviors, neonates and young infants show that they possess rudimentary powers of object perception (Bower, 1974; 1978). Secondly, the infant is innately endowed to distinguish things from persons. Neonates are able, for example, to respond to adult speech with "interactional behavior-temporal synchrony" (a term which denotes the precise synchrony of a listener's movements to the articulatory patterns of a speaker's speech). Some investigators have argued that this ability may be the necessary framework for the development of language (Condon & Sander, 1974; Condon, 1979). But, according to Trevarthan (1980), the form and quality of the face-to-face interactions between mother and infant suggest much more. These interactions consist of cyclical, complementary, actions and reactions which resemble the kind of postural attitudes, facial expressions, lip and tongue movements and other gestures that may be seen between two adult speakers in conversation. Within the first two months after birth a complex *interpersonal* relationship is formed between the infant and the mother which shows that infants have a faculty of *primary intersubjectivity*—"the knowing of persons and oneself in relation to others" (Trevarthan, 1979, p. 56). Trevarthan argues that this intersubjectivity is the central motivator and regulator for language development and for human mental growth in general; it is, for him, the mechanism for generating culture.

Major accomplishments occur during the first year of life. At primary intersubjectivity, the abilities of two- or three-month-old infants described above are exhibited in an either-or manner. *Either* they can engage in communicative activities with people (mostly the mother) *or* they can show rudimentary adaptive behavior to objects; they cannot engage in activities which include people *and* objects at the same time.

Between four to eight months, an increased interest with objects along with much playfulness occurs. During this period the infant is capable of playing with objects alone so that the praxic mode of knowing and using objects becomes elaborated. Infants below six or seven months enjoy mostly "person games" (such as exploring the mother's face, tickling or hiding). After six months, games may include an object: for example, in the presence of another person, the infant may drop an object, watch for the person's response and then laugh; or, the mother may make an object roll, jingle, appear or disappear for his or her infant's delight. For infants who are under nine-months-old, however, objects are usually perceived and used and persons are usually communicated with. That is, intentions about objects and people are expressed separately. At nine months, an important change in human communication occurs. "A deliberately sought sharing of experiences about events and things is achieved for the first time" (Trevarthan & Hubley, 1978, p. 184). This new integration or combination of the infant's interests of physical reality and acts of communication to persons is termed *secondary intersubjectivity* and enables infants to accept persons in a new way (Trevarthan, 1979, 1980; Trevarthan & Hubley, 1978).

Play, as always, provides many opportunities for the mother and infant to interact. The mother's role in these interactions is crucial. She interprets the infant's behavior as an intention to carry out an action or to try to find out about something, and in the process, the child learns what interpretations his efforts evoke and how these may be modified. The infant has already had much practice in the turn-taking format but now in joint action with the mother, s(he) learns to distinguish segments of agent, action, object, recipient. Rules of substitution and reverse order, as well as a form of early deixis, are dealt with and controlled: e.g., the child as recipient of action becomes an agent of action and the mother, previously an agent, now serves as a recipient of her child's action, and the process then begins again (Bruner, 1975a, 1975b). At the same time, these routines also provide the joint attention of common, concrete foci or topics, which when achieved, can be acted or commented upon. These two concepts of attention and action, developed only in mutuality with a speaker of the language, are fundamental to the acquisition of language. According to Bruner (1975a, 1975b) they provide the basis of two universal structural properties of language: all languages reflect topic-comment structure, an underlying feature of attention, which is realized grammatically as subject and predicate; all languages reflect semantic case structure as an organization of action—they contain categories of agent, action, object of action, recipient of action, and so forth.

It is not surprising that the beginnings of language emerge during the last few months of the first year in terms of a interpersonal functional "proto-language" (Halliday, 1975). It consists of idio-syncratic, but very recognizable, stable vocalizations which represent acts of meaning when addressed to the infant's immediate caregivers. These vocalization-meaning pairs, usually accompanied with consistent gestural patterns, are fundamentally pragmatic in that the infant uses them to obtain assistance from others in order to alter his or her environment in various ways. Thus, armed with the rules of action and attention learned at a prelinguistic level and a set of "primitive speech acts" (Dore, 1975), the one-year-old is on the threshold of spoken language.

The Second Phase of Linguistic Development: Consolidation, Diversification and Variation

What has been described in the preceding section has been characterized as the first phase of language development (Wells, 1981). We have seen that the very early language emerging at the end of the first year is usually idiosyncratic and fundamentally pragmatic, its meaning understood only by those who share the infant's familiar routines and activities. As objects and events of the infant's everyday world, and his own and others activities in this environment, become more and more a conversational focus, the young child discovers another important function of language—namely that language can represent or stand for the objects and events which constitute his experience (Wells, 1981).

Previous views which proposed that sensorimotor intelligence—the content, procedures and structures developed as a result of the child's interaction with his or her "object world" (Karmiloff-Smith, 1979)—*alone* could explain the initial acquisition of language that have been drastically revised. Besides being a symbolic system for representing knowledge, language is also a system for communicating and sharing knowledge. Thus, as the earlier discussion has indicated, contemporary views also regard prespeech communication—the content, procedures and structures developed as a result of the child's interactions with his "people world" (Karmiloff-Smith, 1979)—to be an indispensable, and perhaps even the primary prerequisite factor for the development of language. These processes of cognition and communication are complementary and interactive. In fact, Shields (1978), for example, has argued that since a model of human beings acting in a rule-governed social world contains abstract generalizable features just as complicated as those quantifiable characteristics of objects which govern our actions in the material world, a new "cognitive" model which includes personal constructs has to be developed. In the second phase of language development the picture becomes even more complicated. According to Karmiloff-Smith (1979), "language as a problem-space *per se* irrespective of the content of children's utterances and of their semantic intentions" becomes an important constructive factor in development (1979, p. 2). Specific linguistic items or messages become the means for extending the range and complexity of thought and for elaborating the ways in which people communicate with each other. Thus, children's three worlds—the object world, people world, and language world—all interact and influence each other in complex, synergistic ways (Bloom, 1976).

The second phase of language development is marked by consolidation and diversification (Wells, 1979). Although conventional linguistic forms are initially meager, the child manages to be an active participant in conversations involving the variety of events which constitutes his or her everyday life. Toddlers' linguistic strategies, such as the repetition of what they or others have just uttered—formerly considered to be either simple imitation or irrelevant to their linguistic development—now are seen to be a constructive and sophisticated means to initiate and maintain oral discourse (Keenan, 1977; Wells, 1981). Adults with whom young children interact continue to play an important role in developing these conversation skills. As children become more adept as conversationalists they consolidate the early pragmatic skills of communication and in the process pick up the underlying cultural assumptions and uses of language of their community.

Diversification is also seen in young children's learning and controlling a variety of different language registers (Halliday & Hasan, 1976), an obvious mark of developing communicative competence. Children's linguistic choices become adjusted to meet the features of particular social contexts—the setting, the participants and the specific task involved (Halliday & Hasan, 1976; Wells, 1981).

Much of what has been said about children's language has tended to be expressed in terms of production terms. However, most current views have difficulty separating language production from language comprehension. That is, if conversation or oral discourse is the all-important context of language development, the constructive strategies children employ as speakers are, in part, due to their constructive strategies as listeners. No longer is the comprehension of speech seen as a passive process where a listener merely reacts to an incoming speech signal. Instead, "the task of comprehending speech involves the listener in actively searching for cues to guide his interpretation, in the situational context and in past experience as well as in the signal itself" (Wells, 1981, p. 17).

Research on language development represents an attempt to identify, document and understand the regularities of development. However, within such a developmental framework many individual variations have been noted which are also important to consider. In fact, some believe (e.g., Bridges, Sinka & Bridges, 1981; Naremore, 1979; Thoman, 1979; Denenberg, 1979) that the mounting awareness of individual differences in children's language behavior—to be found in all levels of development—and the ways in which these individual differences interact with the complex set of variables in any context in which language is used, demand that present theories and methodologies be reexamined and revised in major ways.

The present discussion cannot survey all the types of variation, nor cover all the theoretical and/or methodological problems of most of the work on variation, much of which has been extremely naive (Wells, 1979). (See Wells, 1979, for an excellent review on this topic.) Children's overt linguistic behavior or their rate or style of development is never the result of one factor, but due to complex interactions among their inherent attributes (sex, intelligence, personality, etc.) and those found in the environment (family structure, social group affiliation, parental child-rearing methods, cultural environment, features of a particular situation, etc.). Three kinds of variation—*style, sex* and *social background* differences—will be briefly described here since they are the ones discussed most consistently in the psycholinguistic literature.

Prelinguistic variation certainly exists and is presently a focus of ongoing research (Thoman, 1979), but usually discussions about individual differences begin in earnest when children's one or two word utterances emerge at the second phase of language development. Bloom, Lightbown, and Hood (1975) noted differing styles of development when the children they were following were at the early stages of structured utterances: the utterances of some children indicated a nominal preference; whereas the utterances of oth-

ers seemed to show a prenominal preference. Nelson (1973) studied the acquisition of eighteen children's first fifty vocabulary
words and also found a style difference which she called a referential (general names) and expressive (personal-social words) preference. Since then Wells (1981) has stated that Nelson has recently
suggested that this difference may go beyond vocabulary—for example, expressive children have the tendency to use pronouns
(rather than nouns), to produce "unanalyzed" phrases (rather than
constructed two-word utterances) and to have clear intonation (but
poor segmental articulation). Whether there exists, in fact, general
style of development still needs to be confirmed. Some children
appear to be referential speakers for the first fifty words, but then
shift to be more like Nelson's expressive children (Bowerman,
1976, cited in Naremore, 1979). Perhaps some children rely more
heavily on prespeech cognition and others predominantly on pre-
speech communication, but all children need a certain amount of
both (Karmiloff-Smith, 1979). Thus, actually the case is a continuum, not a dichotomy. Even in the studies which have supported the
style distinction, many children do not show any strong preference
at all and when a preference is noted, it usually changes from one
context to another (Wells, 1981).

One of the accepted assumptions of variation is that girls are advanced regarding inherent language ability. However, according to
Wells (1979, 1981), the only sex-related differences which do occur are rate rather than style of acquisition and even these differences are usually insignificant. The sex differences that are seen
are usually due to cultural differences. That is, differences occur
because of the ways in which parents treat and talk to boys and
girls, not because of inherent biologically based abilities as language learners.

For example, Wells (1979) has analyzed conversational sequences between parents and their children when the children were
3½-years-old. (See Wells, 1981, for a description of his population
of 128 children and procedures for data collection.) These sequences were classified two ways: (1) whether the conversation
was initiated by the child or by the parent; and, (2) what the context or dominant purpose the conversation fulfilled. Seventy percent of the sequences were initiated by the children and no significant differences existed between boys and girls regarding initiation
or context/purpose. In the remaining thirty percent of sequence,

however, significant sex differences obtained relative to the contexts in which adults (mostly the mother) chose to initiate conversation. The most striking contrasts occurred in the contexts Wells has termed *Play with Adult Participation*—where adults initiated conversation with boys over girls (ratio of 3.5 to 1), and *Helping and Non-Play*—where adults initiated conversation more with girls (ratio of 2 to 1). This analysis suggests that adults seem to emphasize "useful" and domestic activities in their interactions with girls but emphasize more free-ranging exploratory manipulation of the physical environment with boys (Wells, 1979). Certain research (Cherry, 1975; Serbin, 1981) has indicated that similar sex-related expectations can be found in the verbal interactions between teacher and child in early childhood preschool and play settings as well.

Social background is probably the most controversial type of variation which exists in child language research. It has been claimed that children from lower socioeconomic status (SES) or social class (SES and social class are usually treated as if they are equivalent) possess linguistic or cognitive deficits by showing a developmental lag and/or by using a different language code. The code differences are based on Bernstein's theory (1960, 1965) which describes differences of social class in terms of differences in style of acquisition: the middle class develops an exploratory and explicit use of language—an elaborated code; whereas the lower class develops an expressive and implicit use of language—a restricted code. Similar deficit claims regarding social class and language codes or styles have been advanced in the United States as well (Bereiter & Engleman, 1966).

Three major methodological problems have plagued this research. First, many investigators have not had enough linguistic expertise to recognize the difference between immature and nonstandard, dialectal forms. Secondly, researchers have tended to select their samples from the extreme ends of the SES continuum, or have reduced all social variations into two opposing classes with no regard to the variation which exists in each one. Third, the language data have been collected in a limited number of contrived contexts with the researcher frequently present at the time of collection.

In the Bristol project, Wells (1979) has attempted to overcome these methodological problems by:

(a) sampling from a wide range of divisions on a continuum of social class,
(b) sampling from a wide range of the naturally occurring contexts in which speech occurs in the children's daily lives, with no researcher present during the recording, and
(c) treating local dialect forms, when they occur, in the same way as the equivalent standard forms (p. 388).

All of the analyses that have been carried out so far by Wells and his colleagues (1979, 1981) indicate that social background is *not* a strong determinant for either rate or style of language development. This does not mean to say that some of the differences between children in their rate (or style) of development are not the result of their respective social environments. Indeed, the view described here has argued that the social environment is the major means by which language does develop. Instead, what is being argued is that there is no *a priori* reason to believe that language differences among children are based on either class or code (Wells, 1979, 1981). Unfortunately, we continue to reduce all social variation to a dichotomy and continue to suppose that there are major implications for education based upon such binary class and code differences.

The Third Phase of Linguistic Development: Becoming Literate

The third phase of language development is marked by the acquisition of literacy; as reader and writer, the child extends his or her developing communicative competence to include the use of written language.

To become literate, two major insights—that print is meaningful and that written language is different from speech—must be acquired by the child (Smith, 1982a, 1982b). Just as the prelinguistic child had to discover that patterns of sounds expressed meanings before she/he could learn to produce and comprehend spoken language, likewise the preliterate child must realize that patterns of print represent meanings before she/he can learn to read and write. Recent research (cf. Y. Goodman, 1980; Harste, Burke, & Woodward, 1981) has indicated that the roots of the first insight can be found in the preschool preliterate child who generates and tests hypotheses about the meaning of the written language of labels and signs found in his or her everyday world.

Although it is a kind of written language, the *role* of labels and signs (consisting of single words or small groups of words), however, is similar to typical oral or spoken language. Typical oral language is language accompanying action and assumes a particular immediate perceptual environment and a shared or negotiated perspective between speaker(s) and listener(s). It is a collaborative enterprise in which each participant offers, modifies and extends each other's meanings through turn-taking dialogue. Thus, the language of typical conversation—and the print language of labels and signs—are both embedded in and dependent upon the social situation since this situation provides the cues for interpreting the meaning of the language being used. These have been the conversational interactions by which the first two phases of language development have occurred.

In contrast to this "ancillary" role of language, the role of typical written language is "constitutive" (Halliday, 1977). Typical written language functions across space and time—no shared perspective or perceptual environment exists between readers and writers who are usually unknown to each other. Written language is "monologic" since an interacting, turn-taking conversation partner is absent. Moreover, instead of single words or small groups of words which is characteristic of labels and signs, written language involves the production and comprehension of *continous* text. Because written language is necessarily "disembedded" (Donaldson, 1978) from the situation in which it is either being written or read, typical written language—what Smith terms "text"—must provide, and depend upon, by itself, its own relevant context or clues to meaning.

Thus, the second insight involves children realizing the differences which distinguish oral and written language. Many argue that children acquire this second insight only by being read to, by hearing written language read aloud. They argue that if children have extensive repetitive experiences with a wide range of favorite books, they will learn the *conventions* of written language (Smith, 1982a), or to use Holdaway's (1979) terminology, they will develop a "literacy set." Thus, the roots of the second insight can also be found in the preschool preliterate child who has had these shared-book experiences. The exact nature of the preliterate understandings and what role parents play in their children's literacy learning are examined in several current investigations (cf. Bissex, 1980; Taylor, 1983; Snow, 1983; Heath, 1982).

Within the past decade, a focus of attention *from* the level of word or sentence *to* text has been a major paradigm shift in both linguistic (Beaugrande & Dressler, 1981; Dijk, 1977; Grimes, 1972; Halliday & Hasan, 1976) and psychological (Mandler & Johnson, 1977; Meyer, 1975; Rumulhart, 1975) inquiries. Work being done in cognitive psychology, linguistics and artificial intelligence is heavily influencing current theories and research in reading and writing, and, as a result, these two areas have experienced their own paradigm shifts (see Spiro, Bruce, & Brewer, 1980; Smith, 1982a; and Frederiksen & Dominic, 1981; Smith, 1982b; respectively, for recent examples).

Reading is no longer viewed as just the sounding-out of letters or the decoding or recognition of words; writing is more than the forming of letters or the encoding or spelling of words. Reading and writing are considered as cognitive, linguistic, communicative processes by which human, social intentions are expressed and conveyed through the conventions of written language. It is clear that readers and writers—even those who are novices, just entering phase three of language development—are active constructors in these processes; but we have only just begun to explore all that is involved in the composition and comprehension of different written genres, which fulfill various communicative functions or purposes, and we have a long way to go to understand the ways by which readers and writers accomplish such tasks.

Along with the advent of literacy, phase three ushers in a new kind of thinking—the child becomes capable of reflecting on his or her experience and being consciously aware of his or her mental states. Whether the acquisitions of literacy is a cause or facilitator for this new cognitive functioning will not be debated here (see Olson, 1977, and Wells, 1981, for a review of the major arguments), but it is evident that the strong links of language, action and context of situation so characteristic in the earlier two phases must be loosened in order to become literate. In this third phase a new function for language emerges; children begin to see language as an object and this metalinguistic awareness provides them both a new "tool for thinking."

Summary of Contemporary Views on Language Development

The contemporary views on language development as set forth above can be summarized around three major points.

Nature-Nurture

Extreme views on either end of the nature-nurture continuum have been discarded: S-R conditioning cannot account for the creativity seen in the understanding and use of language and wholesale or general innateness of language cannot explain the fact that knowledge or skill is essentially adapted and self-regulating and therefore interactional in origin. Today's view is more of a balanced one and argues that both innate endowment and linguistic environment are necessary (Wells, 1981).

Trevarthan (1979, 1980) believes that the behaviors of infants are indicative of an innateness for social interaction and cooperative understanding. He maintains just as adamantly that these are only *necessary* preconditions or propensities, *not sufficient* ones. These are preadaptations for language or whatever skill or knowledge you have in mind and require complementary elaborate adaptations in the behaviors of mothers or other consistent and affectionate caretakers. Thus, it is *specific* innateness which will be admitted to, not general innateness. Bruner (1980), for example, has argued that the secondary intersubjectivity seen at nine or ten months (when protolanguage emerges) represents "innate ostension" or the infant's predisposing procedures for indicating or bringing a partner's attention to an object or action or state and that this assumption on the part of the child that things and events are shared in the world by others provides a natural basis for developing linguistic reference. Bruner also argues that this first step of intersubjectivity will require interpreting adults to help and support the infant develop control of particular instances or applications of reference. What is also accepted, then, is not a *linguistic* innateness but aspects of humans action and attention, although some researchers (Wells, 1981) are still open to consider that organizational principles specific to linguistic form may require some innate structure or "knowledge" of a language-specific kind.

Language as the Communication of Intentions

Psycholinguists are more willing to talk about "intentions" nowadays. The whole notion of communication presupposes intent or purpose in that any communication succeeds or fails. Thus a communication framework has enabled investigators to incorporate intentions in their developmental theories and explanations way before intentions are realized in linguistic means. Trevarthan (1980) has argued that the regularity of the movements that two-month-old infants display towards objects versus towards humans is evidence for imputing rudimentary "motives" or "intentions" to these movements. Bruner (1975a, 1975b) has maintained that mothers act and talk to their infants *as if* the infants have intentions. Thus, while "intentions" are difficult to deal with and messy to establish, they are assumed by many researchers. They believe that since language use is premised upon presuppositions about intentions, the construct of intentions cannot be avoided and current efforts are being made to operationalize and systematically analyze intentionality (cf. Greenfield, 1980; Morgan & Green, 1980).

Child as Active and Constructive in Learning Language

Closely related to the other two points is the point that children are not passive learners in the course of development. Psycholinguists have managed to overcome the tendency to view the child only from the adult perspective (Lamendella, 1976). Even though a young child may possess few, if any, conventional linguistic forms, she/he can participate, pragmatically speaking, in communicative exchanges. It is obvious that children's systems—what they have integrated about people, the world and language—cannot coincide with adults because children are trying to construct the system from a particular developmental place within it. That is why researchers are more interested now in looking at how some aspect of language—for example, noun determiners—gradually change *function* from the child's point of view rather than when it appears in a child's language (Karmiloff-Smith, 1979). There is an acknowledgement of activities such as strategies, processes, patterns by which children manage to construct rule systems to generate appropriate communicative utterances which allow for variation—there may be more than one way for children to arrive at a given structure or meaning (Naremore, 1979).

RELATING LANGUAGE DEVELOPMENT
TO BRAIN DEVELOPMENT

Now that we have sketched out some important notions of language development, we are confronted with the task of outlining how brain tissue is organized and/or grows to support or create this language development. It is important to warn at the outset that despite the especially active brain research of the past two decades, biological theories within which language data can be interpreted are not forthcoming. That is, the chronic problem of biology—the relationship between structure and function—remains. As Colby (1977) states: "The conceptual distance between symbolic rules and neurons is so great that it is difficult to propose how knowledge about one might contribute to knowledge of the other" (p. 7). We have made the problem much worse by constantly making conceptual mistakes, by simplifying issues which are very complex, and by deluding ourselves into believing that we know something about the biology of language acquisition when it is very clear that we do not.

The following discussion will review major areas in which language function and the brain have been investigated. The first few sub-sections will focus mainly on research which has involved adults. They, however, will provide important background for the later sub-sections which will more specifically address developmental issues.

Morphological Hemispheric Asymmetries

Most discussions about language and the brain begin by noting the relationship between the left cerebral hemisphere and language functions. As early as 1861, Broca presented the cases of two patients who had loss of speech and also had a lesion or injury in the region of the third frontal convolution of the left hemisphere. Later in 1874, Wernicke described a kind of language impairment different from Broca's called sensory aphasia where patients demonstrated paraphasia, word-finding and language comprehension symptoms. These latter difficulties again involved the left hemisphere but in a different spot; namely, the posterior superior portion of the first temporal gyrus.

Today there is little doubt that the integrity of Broca's area, Wernicke's area and parts of the left parietal lobe, including especially the angular gyrus, are crucial for normal linguistic functioning in most adults. What has been added to this picture in the last decade or so is the finding that anatomical or morphological asymmetries of the human brain are also associated with some of the classical speech areas (Geschwind & Levitsky, 1968). The most frequently mentioned finding is that the planum temporale is generally larger in the left hemisphere than in the right in both adult and infant brains (Wada, 1977; Witelson & Pallie, 1973). Based on this finding, Witelson (1977) and others have argued that this larger left planum temporale reflects the usual functional dominance of the left hemisphere for language.

Whitaker and Ojemann (1977) have reviewed the asymmetries in various paired structures of the human body, however, and have argued that if one considers other regions of the brain (and the rest of the body as well, but the present account will be limited to the areas of the brain) that are part of the speech and language system, the picture is not at all clear. There are several areas which are larger in the right hemisphere: the Heschl's gyrus, Broca's area, and the superior temporal gyrus, the posterior part of which is the major part of Wernicke's area. Thus, it is reasonable to conclude, as Whitaker and Ojemann (1977) have, that it is "unwise to associate language per se with consistent left-greater-than-right differences of only one portion of the cortical language areas" (p. 460). Perhaps if we knew the exact role of the planum temporale performs compared to the superior temporal gyrus, then maybe the morphological asymmetries might be more interpretable. Unfortunately, we have as yet no idea what roles these areas play in language (Whitaker & Ojemann, 1977; Ojemann, 1983).

There are also major problems in measuring these classical speech-related landmarks in the human brain which are so complex and variable (Marshall, 1980). Many authorities even disagree as to where the angular gyrus really is: some place it in the posterior part of the temporal lobe; some place it in the parietal lobe (Ojemann, 1977; Marshall, 1980). Thus, it is risky business indeed to believe that size or place of a biological structure (even if it is present at infancy) in and of itself can provide us with any answers about children's acquisition of the principles of universal grammar.

Commissurotomy Studies

Split-brain patients (those patients who have had the commissures connecting their left and right hemispheres cut in order to control intractable epileptic seizures that cannot be controlled by drug therapy) have been subjects of numerous research studies addressing the nature of lateralization of functions in the cerebral hemispheres. Although their corpus callosums have been severed, these patients are relatively unaffected in ordinary everyday activities. Only under very controlled experimental conditions, however, can specified and limited amounts of information be directed to a patient's one hemisphere to the exclusion of the other. For the most part, the general finding of the studies have indicated that the left hemisphere is better at, or in control of, analytic, sequential and linguistic tasks, whereas the right hemisphere appeared to be involved with nonlinguistic, holistic or Gestalt functioning (see Springer & Deutsch, 1981, and Segalowitz, 1983, for recent reviews of this research).

In the 1970s researchers, especially Zaidel (1978, 1979), began to argue that some findings of split-brain studies provided evidence that the disconnected right-hemisphere is also active in certain aspects of linguistic-related processes. According to Whitaker and Ojemann (1977), however, conclusions of these kind of studies had led to generalizations about the left and right brain which are premature. Since it is not always clear as to what specific hypothesis is being entertained in many of the commissurotomy studies, they consider three possible ones. If the hypothesis is that the right hemisphere (RH) might be able to support a level of linguistic function superficially comparable to that of the left, hemidecordicate subjects (those patients who have had one hemisphere—the left in this case—removed in infancy to control intractable seizures) have already answered this in the affirmative. If the hypothesis is that the RH might be able to support any linguistic function, what we know about global aphasia has positively answered that. If the hypothesis is that there is an "X" amount of linguistic ability in the RH under normal circumstances, then these split-brain studies are not going to provide the answers.

Inferences are frequently made about the functions of the LH and RH, as well as the corpus callosum itself, yet no information is provided about the location or extent of previous lesions (i.e., noncallosal) in the brains of these patients. The fact that these patients have had seizures for a long time suggest that there may have been many opportunities for their brains to functionally reorganize. Moreover, there are two aspects about the operation itself which underlines the uniqueness of these patients. First, even the surgeon is unable to know how much of the corpus callosum was cut, how much was spared, or how large (or small) the remaining minor commissures are (Segalowitz, 1983). Secondly, sometimes one of the hemispheres sustains damage in the process of getting to the corpus callosum (Segalowitz, 1983; Whitaker & Ojemann, 1977). That is, the surgical approach to the corpus callosum to be cut is done through the nondominant hemisphere (usually the RH), and when the mesial surface is retracted to expose the corpus callosum, sometimes this damages the mesial surface of the opposite hemisphere. For all of the above reasons, Whitaker and Ojemann (1977) conclude that "the callosum-sectioned patients do not seem to be a suitable population in which to study the normal linguistic abilities of the RH" (p. 461). It is reasonable to expand this statement and argue that it is faulty thinking to infer or generalize any aspect of cognitive functioning of normal, intact brains based upon the left- and right-sided skills demonstrated by a very small number of split-brain patients. Yet, this research, more than any other, has been responsible for the continuation of simple dichotomies—the left hemisphere processes language tasks, the right hemisphere processes nonlinguistic tasks—and for outlandish extrapolations for normal functioning. More will be said about this issue of generalization in subsequent sub-sections and in the implications section.

Behavioral Hemispheric Asymmetries in Normals

Sparked by the left-right dichotomies seen in the split-brain studies, many studies during the past two decades have investigated lateralization or asymmetric hemispheric functioning of normal subjects. Various techniques were adopted to study the relative abilities of each hemisphere on specific tasks. One set of techniques—e.g., the dichotic listening task and the visual half-filled technique—relies on the fact that senses like hearing and seeing involve major contralateral connections. Other techniques attempt to tap brain functioning by examining correlates of brain activity—electrical patterns as recorded by an electroencephalograph (EEG techniques) and the amount of blood flowing to various regions of the brain cerebral blood flow (CBF) techniques.

Visual and Auditory Asymmetries

Many of the dichotic and tachistoscopic half-filled studies have centered upon the verbal-nonverbal distinction. Investigators have made simplistic assumptions that ear or eye advantage indicates language or nonlanguage representation on the opposite side. That is, when stimuli such as words or single letters or syllables, etc., show a right-side advantage (i.e., the stimuli in a right visual field or in the right ear are more accurately or more quickly identified), it is evidence of left-hemisphere specialization for language functions; when nonverbal stimuli (like dots or faces) show a left-side advantage, it is indicative of right-hemisphere functioning. Both techniques have been used with children and unfortunately just as simplistic assumptions regarding the *degree* of lateralization, based upon findings of *degree* of asymmetry, have been made. More will be said about this issue in a later sub-section.

Baffling inconsistencies and many problems exist in the dichotic and tachistoscopic studies (Kinsbourne, 1979; Marshall, 1980; Segalowitz, 1983; Springer & Deutsch, 1981). A major problem is one of reliability—that is, subjects frequently may show a right-ear advantage for some speech stimulus during testing in one week but shift to a left-ear advantage for the same stimuli a week later. Another major problem is that people appear to adopt strategies (not under the control of the experimenter) in the way they attend to, treat, or report about, stimuli, all of which may affect their ear or eye advantage. Finally, even though one would expect that dichotic and visual measures of verbal stimuli, for example, would be measuring the same lateralized function, these tests are not highly correlated (Springer & Deutsch, 1981).

Physiological Correlates of Function

Psychophysiological techniques more directly measure brain activity and therefore bypass the need for many assumptions that are made in the dichotic listening and visual half-filled tasks. As will be noted later, these measures unfortunately have their own conceptual and methodological problems. However, since they study relationships between brain activity during behavior, they have been responsible for drastically altering exaggerated dichomotized claims about left-right asymmetries. There is little evidence in the psychophysiological studies to support the notion that either one hemisphere or the other "turns on" to perform a specific task all by itself. All of the measures indicate the involvement of many areas of the brain in even the simplest task. Moreover, while asymmetries in activity between hemispheres based on these techniques do exist, they can normally be extremely subtle, thereby keeping us from conceiving of hemispheric specialization in overly simple terms.

EEG Techniques

Of the EEG techniques, two are the most popular: EEG alpha waves and evoked potentials (EP)—sometimes also called event-related potentials (ERP) or average evoked responses (AER). A twofold assumption underlies the examination of alpha waves that increased alpha waves in a given area indicate general "arousal," that is, a brain "resting," not processing information in that area, and that *decreased* alpha waves in a given area indicate that the opposite, that is, that part of the brain is actively processing information. Using such a paradigm, putatively "left hemisphere" tasks, such as speaking, listening, reading, writing (both copying text and generating text) and arithmetic, and "right hemisphere" tasks, such as block design, mirror tracking, etch-a-sketch, etc., have been studied and have found asymmetry effects (Galin, 1979). With respect to the "language" tasks, however, individual language tasks can show different characteristic patterns of hemispheric engagement. For example, when right-handed subjects have been involved with three tasks—speaking, reading and a block design task—they show relatively greater right hemisphere participation in reading than in speaking, but less than in the spatial block construction (Galin, 1979). As already mentioned, results such as these guard against viewing left-right hemispheric functioning in terms of a simple dichotomy. Galin's (1979) warning is as follows:

> The important point to stress here is that there is no verbal task which is "representative" of "language"; patterns of hemispheric engagement in reading differ from the pattern of speaking or writing. Any single test used to assess "language lateralization," such as tachistoscopic presentation of words to be read in each hemifield, or dichotic listening, is likely to mislead by over simplifying (p. 137).

The use of EEG alpha activity as an index of lateral specialization, however, has its own host of problems. First of all, there is no general agreement as to which neuropsychological functions are being tapped by alpha activity. Alpha activity can be increased (augmented) or decreased (blocked) by changes in attention, arousal or anxiety (Orne & Paskewitz, 1974), and can show much individual difference during the same task (Orne & Wilson, 1971), all of which questions whether alpha activity is indexing cognition functioning at all. In addition, it is possible that brainstem or thalamic processes may be superimposing their effects on alpha activity so that observed alpha asymmetry may not solely be due to cerebral functioning but due instead to also subcortical activities. Moreover, just as in the dichotic listening and visual half-field task studies, related problems of strategy effects are also seen in EEG studies (Beaumont, Mayes, & Rugg, 1978).

The major advantage the EEG alpha index has is that it can assess more naturalistic cognitive activities like speaking, reading or writing, yet, this advantage itself simultaneously represents a disadvantage. The fact that the index is an overall continous measure also means that it is not sensitive to various individual events which make up the speaking, reading or writing process. It is the other EEG method, the evoked potential (EP), which is supposedly better able to deal with specific events (Donchin & McCarthy, 1979). However, this technique is an averaged measure of brain activity and requires transient repetition of the same stimulus. For this reason, the stimuli used in EP studies tend to be isolated "bits" of language such as consonant stops or words. More recently, some studies have placed word stimuli in short seven-word sentences in the hope that these tasks will be more like natural language processing (Kutas & Hillyard, 1980, 1982). Nevertheless, a subject's behavior in an EP study is one of responding to single words flashed one at a time on a screen, for example, and that is very different from ordinary reading—namely, making sense of connected prose by serial fixations and targeted eye movements.

Choosing to use one or the other EEG technique, therefore, is much like choosing to be between a rock and a hard place. In addition, both techniques have to contend with the "thorny" problem of anatomical asymmetries (Galin, 1979). That is, in lateralization studies investigators compare activity in a particular region in one hemisphere with the corresponding area in the other hemisphere. This is accomplished by placing electrodes on the scalp of each hemisphere with strict adherence to an assumption of hemisphere symmetry. However, as already pointed out, some areas of the brain are larger (or smaller) in one hemisphere than the other; moreover, many individual differences exist (Whitaker & Selnes, 1977; Ojemann, 1983). Consequently, differences of left-right hemisphere activities observed in these studies may not be due to functional differences at all; they may be merely due to electrode placement differences.

Cerebral Blood-Flow Techniques

The method of measuring regional cerebral blood flow (CBF) is based on the fact that the flow of blood through the tissues of the body varies with the level of metabolism and functional activity in those tissues. That is, as areas of the cortex are activated during a particular task, more metabolic effort is expended, and more blood is required. Blood flow is measured by detecting the radioactivity in the blood (the result of an injection or inhalation of radioactive xenon). These data are analyzed by a computer and then projected to a screen where different colors can depict and differentiate relative percentages of blood flow increases in various parts of the cerebral cortex. Even more than electrophysiological measures, measures of CBF have demonstrated how much complex behavioral processes involve active participation of many areas of *both* left and right hemispheres.

Some hemisphere differences have been observed, for example, when subjects perform a verbal analogy test versus a nonverbal perceptual test (Risberg, Halsey, Wills, & Wilson, 1975), but these differences are very subtle. The most consistent and impressive finding has been that different processes such as speaking, reading aloud and silent reading are carried out by several circumscribed cortical regions brought into action in different but specific patterns and that both the right and left hemispheres become active in much the same manner (Lassen, Ingvar, & Skinhoj, 1978). Speaking aloud activates the following three areas in both hemispheres: the auditory cortex, the face, tongue and mouth areas of the somatosensory and motor cortex, and the upper premotor cortex (which includes supplementary motor area); as well as Broca's area in the lower part of the left frontal lobe and the corresponding part of the right frontal lobe. Reading aloud activates three more areas in both hemispheres—the visual association cortex, the frontal eye fields and the primary visual cortex—so that seven discrete cortical regions become simultaneously involved. The contrast between reading aloud and silent reading is extremely interesting. During silent reading two areas—the mouth areas of the somatosensory cortex and motor cortex and the auditory areas—are not activated, although the five other areas are active. Thus, when we read silently we do not need to "mouth" the words of text (remember the somatosensory or motor cortex is not active) nor do we need to "hear" the words as we read (no auditory cortex activation). This latter finding regarding silent reading seriously questions many commonplace notions and certain theories of reading. Lassen et al. (1978) were surprised to find so much activation in the homologous area of Broca's area in the right hemisphere during speaking, since loss of speech is seen so consistently only when lesions occur in that area in the left hemisphere. Further investigations have suggested some discernible differences between the left and right hemisphere speakers: "in the left hemisphere an increase in flow is usually seen in the mouth area and the auditory cortex separately, whereas in the right hemisphere the two often form one confluent active region. Moreover, the supplementary motor area in left hemisphere is usually more active during speech than the one in the right hemisphere" (Lassen et al., 1978, p. 70). Again when hemisphere differences occur, they appear to be very subtle ones. The supplementary motor area activation in speaking, and in reading aloud and silent reading has been observed in all voluntary movements and Lassen et al., believe that this area is involved in the planning of sequential motor tasks, but whether differences exist between the left and right hemisphere in the supplementary motor area in the two reading processes like those suggested in speaking is unknown.

Cerebral blood-flow techniques also have limitations as measures of brain activity. Current systems show mostly cortical patterns and do not provide accurate information about the deepest regions of the brain (Springer & Deutsch, 1981). Since many current theories and research on language acquisition and processing include prominent subcortical involvement (Penfield & Roberts, 1959; Lamendella, 1976; Pribram, 1976; Ojemann, 1983), techniques are needed so that activity in deeper parts can also be analyzed. In addition, blood flow is probably not responsive enough to rapid variations in brain activity, although more sophisticated techniques to monitor and measure these kinds of variations are being developed (Springer & Deutsch, 1981). Finally, blood-flow techniques have their own methodological problems. A "cross-talk effect" (a partial recording of radiation originating in the contralateral hemisphere), which can underestimate true hemispheric flow asymmetries, and other such difficulties also arise in the use of

CBF techniques (Risberg, 1980) and these must be considered when interpreting the findings of these studies.

Developmental Lateralization

The traditional view of language lateralization—"progressive lateralization" (Kinsbourne, 1979; Woods, 1980)—was first set forth by Lennenberg (1967). Based on his analysis of clinical case studies, Lennenberg concluded that: (1) any aphasia resulting from lateralized cerebral damage is milder and more quickly recovered the younger the child is; (2) aphasia resulting from lesions in the *right* hemisphere is more common the younger the child is. From these conclusions, he argued that language lateralization is completed at puberty and is the end point of a developmental process in which initially both hemispheres are equally involved in language acquisition. Krashen (1973) has supported the progressive lateralization hypothesis in a similar way but suggests that the process is completed much earlier, at five- or six-years-old.

Findings which have indicated that the degree of asymmetry increases with increasing age of the child in a number of dichotic and visual hemifield studies is also consistent with the progressive lateralization hypothesis (Satz, 1975). By assuming there is a one-to-one correspondence between asymmetry of performance and degree of functional lateralization of language, investigators have inferred that these cross-sectional studies are evidence that the older the child, the more language is lateralized.

Various reasons have been advanced to "explain" the progress of lateralization. Marshall (1979) has summarized the major ones: "The left hemisphere matures faster than the right; the right hemisphere's linguistic abilities atrophy; the development of right-handedness (either genetically preprogrammed or taught) 'induces' greater skill in the left hemisphere control of speech; the left hemisphere inhibits the right hemisphere's capacities for language via cortico-cortico and cortico-subcortical pathways" (p. 446). An implicit implication of the progression of left language lateralization is that it is "good." This has led many to question the lateralization of language of any population who did not show this "normal" progress of asymmetry—women, non-right handers, children of lower socioeconomic status, and some pathological groups (Kinsbourne, 1979). Findings of such "atypical" lateralization have usually been based on hand, foot, eye and ear preference or on dichotic listening or split visual scores. Both of these sources of evidence, however, are highly suspect. Kinsbourne (1979) states that preference does not give any reliable information about language lateralization; Marshall (1979) argues that there is no evidence that left handedness or motoric ambilaterality is intrinsically pathological, nor is it in any way associated with either verbal or visuospatial difficulties. A similar situation regarding the dichotic listening and visual half-field studies exists. Because of the lack of control of a range of mediating variables in these studies—the nature of the signal, task difficulty, a subject's efficiency and motivation, a subject's cognitive style or mental set, the physical asymmetry of the laboratory in which tests are administered, to mention a few (Kinsbourne, 1979)—no reliable relationship obtains between cerebral lateralization, as indexed by dichotic listening or visual half-freed scores, and the acquisition of effective speech or effective reading (Kinsbourne, 1979; Marshall, 1979).

During the last decade, the progressive lateralization thesis has been seriously challenged in other ways to the point that it is even reasonable to accept the null hypothesis—cerebral dominance for language does not develop (Kinsbourne, 1979; Marshall, 1979, 1980). Evidence has been presented from several sources to support the view that ultimate lateralization characteristics exist in the same form from the beginning—"invariant lateralization" (Kinsbourne, 1979). Part of this evidence is the observation that morphological asymmetries (favoring the left) associated with the classical speech areas are present at birth. We have already noted that greater-right-than-left asymmetries also exist and that no morphological asymmetry proves functional asymmetry. Use of electrophysiological techniques with infants have also provided some evidence: Molfese and Molfese (1979) and Molfese (1983) have indicated that some asymmetric EP patterns for certain aspects of speech perception seen in adults can be seen in the very young infants; and, Wada (1977) has reported the asymmetric EP coherence measures of checks and flashes for infants are similar to those obtained for adults. Although these findings do support the notion that cerebral dominance does *not develop,* it is important to note that we are far from understanding *what* is lateralized in the infant (Marshall, 1979; Wada, 1977).

Finally, contrary to Lennenberg's earlier formulations, more recent scrutiny of clinical cases has argued that even in very early childhood an injury in the left hemisphere is likely to have a deleterious effect on a child's language (Marshall, 1979; Woods, 1980). Thus, the answer to the question, "Is it better to have your brain lesion early?" is no longer an unqualified "yes." The results of animal studies have indicated that answers can never be a simple yes or no. Depending on the site of the lesion and when it is incurred, the behavioral consequences can be functional sparing—nearly complete or very partial—a retardation, or even a bizarre abnormality (Schneider, 1979). We have not done the longitudinal studies in child aphasia to know any definite answers about the plasticity or equipotentiality of the infant and child brain or to know even what types of symptoms an injured brain might display at different maturational stages (Marshall, 1979).

The traditional theory of progressive lateralization has been questioned, but what has the challenge explained? It is doubtful that crude dichotomies so characteristic of the lateralization literature will be helpful in understanding the acquisition of language although there is some trend recently to treat the question of cerebral dominance as a nonissue (Kirk, 1983); that is, to avoid any discussion concerning the presence or absence of hemispheric differences and to focus instead more on the fundamental nature of the process (Molfese, 1983).

Brain Growth

If the area of lateralization does not seem to be that promising for providing answers or exaplanations regarding language acquisition, let us follow the current fad and "go back to the basics" and consider neuronal growth. This area of brain is always appealing since it is so reasonable to assume that the nervous system must have attained some degree of structural maturity in order to support and sustain a process as complex as language acquisition. The human brain shows more elaborated brain structure before birth than any other animal; moreover, the human brain has more intricate postnatal differentiations than any other animal (Rose, 1980; Trevarthan, 1983). It doubles its volume during the first year of infancy and attains about 90% of its adult volume by the age of three (Trevarthan, 1983). Accompanying this dramatic change in physical size are equally dramatic changes in the child's capabilities in language (and in other domains as well). Are these physical and functional changes coincidences? In what ways can changes in the infant and child brain provide us with the answers and explanations we seek about language development?

One of the most popular parameters of neuronal growth is axonal myelination. Using histological methods, it has been possible to trace the chronology of myelination in different regions and fiber systems of the brain (Yakovlev & Lecours, 1967; Lecours, 1975). Lecours (1975) has described the myelogentic cycle of a particular area of the brain as follows:

the *myllogentic cycle* of a given fiber system or region is (sic) the period extending from the time of the first appearance of stainable myelin sheath in that system or region to the age when tinctorial intensity shows no further visually discernible gain when compared with the same system or region in the (normal) brain of a 28-year-old adult....(p. 122).

Lecours has further claimed that these cycles "reflect the functional maturation of the brain and therefore can be related to the emergence and gradual differentiation in man of behavioral patterns such as locomotion, manipulation of instruments, articulated speech, and language" (p. 122).

The correspondences Lecours and others (cf. Trevarthan, 1983) have drawn on brain structure and function are interesting, but they remain correspondences. That is, as correlations, neither causes nor necessary preconditions can be inferred from them (Marshall, 1979; 1980). For example, according to Lecours, the post-thalamic pathways to the auditory cortex show a relatively late onset of myelination and a long, slow progress of completion. From this, should we infer that the auditory capabilities of the infant are minimal? Certainly not, for much of the data which has been advanced to challenge the progressive lateralization thesis has demonstrated the opposite—for example, that two-month old infants are sensitive to many place-of-articulation differences (Jusczyk & Thompson, 1978) and that neonates respond to the articulatory patterns of adult speech with "interactional behavior-temporal synchrony" (Condon, 1979), and so forth. What can be claimed based on these data, then, is "either that myelination is (relatively) unimportant for effective conduction of impulses to the auditory cortex or that thalamic nuclei can mediate subtle perceptual differences" (Marshall, 1979, p. 451).

Thus there is no way in which straightforward inferences can be made from the physiological domain to the psychological domain. This is the case for axonal myelination and it is the case also for dendritic arborization, the other popular parameter of neuronal growth. Again, it is not possible to deduce that a particular density of cortical synapses is required before a particular behavior of function may emerge (Marshall, 1979). Researchers actually operate in the opposite fashion. They interpret (or infer) structured based upon what they know about function. Trevarthan (1983) is a recent example of this procedure. He has noted the behaviors displayed by infants at two months and nine months (primary and secondary intersubjectivity, respectively) and then has attempted to interpret what we know about neuron production and the plan of their migration into the neocortex (Sedman & Radic, 1973), the differentiation or elaboration of nerve cells or synapse formation (Dobbing & Smart, 1974; Sedman & Radic, 1973), the course of myelination (Lecours, 1975), and other aspects of structure to account for those infant behaviors. However, Trevarthan (1983) admits himself, that the evidence he has offered "cannot specify the anatomy of an 'interjectivity mechanism'" (p. 76). At best his endeavor represents a *hypothesis* of a cerebral system for regulating growth and cooperative understanding.

IMPLICATIONS FOR EDUCATION

It is difficult to suggest educational implications based on conclusions about the relationship between language development and brain development when it is clear that very little information about the relationship exists. Nothing in the brain research provides any answers as to how developing brain structures sustain the protolanguage seen at the end of an infant's first year, or the ways by which young children learn to use language appropriately in different communicative contexts, including those contexts in which the medium of written language is prominent. We have found that sometimes infant brains have the same bumps that adult brains have and that certain stimuli elicit the same evoked potentials in infant brains as they do in adult brains, but we have no idea what these findings mean for explaining any aspect of the process by which children learn language. We have no principled ideas about how language is coded by the brain and therefore we cannot specify the ways by which social or environmental forces might affect that "code." We have learned about neurones, synapses, transmitter substances and patterns of connectivity in the language areas but we do not know whether they differ in any important respects from those characteristic in other parts of the brain.

Since it is easier to do, let us first specify implications for education which are *not* warranted by brain research. First and foremost no decisions about instruction or curriculum should be made based on the lateralization literature. Suggestions such as those offered by Chall and Mirsky (1978) have been influential:

...there are suggestions to strengthen the "weak" left-hemisphere processes by using more the intact right hemisphere for learning of left-hemisphere processes...Reading comprehension improves by teaching students to visual and use imagery, which presumably are right-hemisphere capabilities.

...A second recommendation is that students who are weak in academic skills (based heavily on the left hemisphere) be taught music, construction, and other activities in order to provide these right-brained children with some activities in which they can excel....

...They need "right-brained" activities to give them a sense of success and self-worth....(p. 374).

These implications for education are based on simplistic notions of left-right hemispheric functioning and are extremely misleading. This is not to say that reading comprehension might be facilitated by helping students use imagery or that a well-rounded curriculum might provide a better education for children. What is absurd is to base these educational decisions on studies of lateralization whose findings have been inconsistent, fraught with conceptual and methodological difficulties, and still remain controversial (cf. Puccetti, 1981, with its open commentary and Gazzaniga, 1981, with responses by Levy & Zaidel). Even Segalowitz (1983), a prominent investigator in the field has warned: "It very well may be that a diverse curriculum with some emphasis in nonverbal skills leads to a better-educated child. However, the argument in favor of a well-rounded education should not invoke lateralization" (p. 207).

Making decisions on educational policy and practice based on brain growth is also misconceived. Epstein (1978), for example, has claimed that "brain development stages may well manifest themselves in correlated, if not causally related, stages of mental development" (p. 344). Brain development means axonal myelination and dentritic arborization, and mental development means Piagetian stages in Epstein's thesis. Again what we have are merely correlations; in no way are these correspondences causally related. Many social, linguistic and contextual factors affect what children do in Piagetian tasks (Donaldson, 1978; Carmi, 1981; Karmiloff-Smith, 1979), so it is dangerous to suggest that their performance is somehow directly related to size of their brains. Again, the recommendation that educational strategies and curriculum planning should be decided upon developmental grounds is applauded; what is not useful is to base that recommendation on brain growth.

What, then, are reasonable implications for education based upon recent brain research? Practically every technique which has been used to examine the relationship between language and the brain has indicated that subjects are *active* in processing the tasks they are asked to perform—they frequently adopt strategies which are not under the control of the experimenter—and that substantial *individual differences* exist. What is suggested, therefore, is *not* to view children as passive learners or as empty receptacles in which to pour in "facts of language." This is inconsistent with the brain research findings. Instead, what is recommended is to realize and appreciate that children are constructive learners and to make decisions about instruction based upon what strategies individual children employ in learning and using language. Of course, this has always been good educational practice. Speculation about the brain structures of the learner will not make that practice any better!

REFERENCES

Beaugrande, R. de, & Dressler, W. *Introduction to text linguistics,* Longman, 1981.

Beaumont, J., Mayes, A. R., & Rugg, M. D. Asymmetry in EEG alpha coherence and power: Effects of task and sex: *Electroencephalography and Clinical Neurophysiology,* 1978, *45,* 393–401.

Bellugi, U. *The acquisition of negation.* Unpublished doctoral dissertation, Harvard University, 1967.

Bellugi-Klima, U. Linguistic mechanisms underlying child speech. In E. Zale (Ed.), *Proceedings of the conference on language and language behavior.* New York: Appleton-Century-Crofts, 1968.

Bereiter, C., & Engleman, S. *Teaching disadvantaged children in the pre-school.* Englewood Cliffs, N. J.: Prentice-Hall, 1966.

Berko, J. The child's learning of English morphology. *Word,* 1958, *14,* 150-177.

Bernstein, B. Language and social class. *British Journal of Sociology.* 1960, *11,* 261-276.

Bernstein, B. A sociolinguistic approach to social learning. In J. Gould (Ed.), *Penguin survey of the social sciences.* Harmondsworth, Middlesex: Penguin Books, 1965.

Bissex, G. L. GNYS AT WRK: *A child learns to write and read.* Cambridge: Harvard University Press, 1980.

Bloom, L. *Language development: Form and function in emerging grammars.* Cambridge, Mass: M. I. T. Press, 1970.

Bloom, L. An integrated perspective on language development. *Papers and Reports on Child Language Development,* Department of Linguistics, Stanford University, 1976, *12,* 1-22.

Bloom, L., Rocissano, L., & Hood, L. Adult-child discourse: Developmental interaction between information processing and linguistic knowledge. *Cognitive Psychology,* 1976, *8,* 521-552.

Bloom, L., Lightbown, P., & Hood, L. Structure and variation in child language. *Monographs of the Society for Research in Child Development,* 1975, *40.*

Bower, T. G. R. *Development in infancy.* San Francisco: Freeman & Co., 1974.

Bower, T. G. R. Perceptual development: object and space. In E. C. Carterette and M. P. Friedman (Eds.), *Handbook of perception, vol. 8.* New York: Academic Press, 1978.

Bridges, A., Sinha, C., & Walkerdine, V. The development of comprehension. In G. Wells (Ed.), *Learning through interaction: The study of language development.* Cambridge: Cambridge University Press, 1981.

Brown, R. *A first language: The early stages.* Cambridge, Mass.: Harvard University Press, 1973.

Bruner, J. S. The ontogenesis of speech acts. *Journal of Child Language,* 1975a, *2,* 1-19.

Bruner, J. S. From communication to language—A psychological perspective. *Cognition,* 1975b, *3,* 255-287.

Bruner, J. S. Afterword. In D. R. Olson (Ed.), *The social foundations of language and thought.* New York: W. W. Norton & Co., 1980.

Carmi, G. The role of context in cognitive development. *The Quarterly Newsletter of the Laboratory of Comparative Human Cognition,* 1981, *3,* 46-54.

Chafe, W. L. *Meaning and the structure of language.* Chicago: The University of Chicago Press, 1970.

Chall, J. S., & Mirsky, A. F. The implications for education. In J. S. Chall & A. F. Mirsky (Eds.), *Education and the brain.* Chicago: National Society for the Study of Education, 1978.

Cherry, L. Teacher-child verbal interaction: An approach to the study of sex differences. In B. Thorne & N. Henley (Eds.), *Language and sex: Difference and dominance.* Rowley, Mass: Newburg House, 1975.

Chomsky, C. *The acquisition of syntax in children from 5 to 10.* Cambridge, Mass: The M. I. T. Press, 1969.

Chomsky, N. A review of *Verbal behavior* by B. F. Skinner. Language, 1959, *35,* 26-58.

Chomsky, N. *Aspects of the theory of syntax.* Cambridge, Mass: M. I. T. Press, 1965.

Clark, E. V. What's in a word? On the child's acquisition of semantics in his first language. In T. E. Moore (Ed.), *Cognitive development and the acquisition of language.* New York: Academic Press, 1973.

Condon, W. S. Neonatal entrainment and enculturation. In M. Bullowa (Ed.), *Before speech: The beginning of interpersonal communication.* Cambridge: Cambridge University Press, 1979.

Condon, W. S., & Sander, L. S. Neonate movement is synchronized with adult speech. *Science,* 1974, *183,* 99-101.

Colby, K. M. Mind models: An overview of current work. *Mathematical Bio-Sciences,* 1978, 159-185.

Denenberg, V. H. Dilemmas and designs for developmental research. In C. L. Ludlow & M. E. Doran-Quine (Eds.), *The neurological bases of language disorders in children: Methods and directions for research.* NINCDS Monograph No. 22. NIH Publication No. 79-440, 1979.

Dobbing, J., & Smart, J. L. Vulnerability of developing brain and behavior. *British Medical Bulletin,* 1974, *30,* 164-168.

Donaldson, M. *Children's minds.* Glasgow: William Collins Sons & Co., Ltd., 1978.

Donchin, E., & McCarthy, G. Event-related brain potentials in the study of cognitive processes. In C. L. Ludlow & M. E. Doran-Quine (Eds.), *The neurological bases of language disorders in children: Methods and directions for research.* NINCDS Monograph No. 22. NIH Publication No. 79-440, 1979.

Dore, J. A pragmatic description of early language learning development. *Journal of Psycholinguistic Research,* 1974, *4,* 343-350.

Dore, J. Holophrases, speech acts and language universals, *Journal of Child Language,* 1975, *2,* 21-40.

Epstein, H. Growth Spurts During Brain Development: Implications for Educational Policy. In J. Chall (Ed.), *Education and the Brain.* Chicago: National Society for the Study of Education, 1978.

Fillmore, C. J. The case for case. In E. Bach & R. T. Harms (Eds.), *Universals in linguistic theory.* New York: Holt, Rinehart and Winston, 1968.

Frederiksen, C. H., & Dominic, J. F. (Eds.) *Writing. The nature, development, and teaching of written communication.* Hillsdale, N. J.: Lawrence Erlbaum Associates, 1981.

Galin, D. EEG studies of lateralization of verbal processes. In C. L. Ludlow & M. E. Doran-Quine (Eds.), *The neurological bases of Language disorders in children. Methods and directions for research.* NINCDS Monograph No. 22. NIH Publication No. 79-440, 1979.

Gazzaniga, M. S. Right hemisphere language following brain bisection: A 20-year perspective (with responses by Levy and Zaidel), *American Psychologist,* 1983, —, 525–549.

Geschwind, N., & Levitsky, W. Human brain, left-right asymmetries in temporal speech regions. *Science,* 1968, *161,* 186-187.

Goodman, Y. M. The roots of literacy. In M. P. Douglass, (Ed.), *Proceedings, Claremont Reading Conference, 44th Annual Yearbook,* Claremont, Ca., 1980.

Greenfield, P. M. Toward an operational and logical analysis of intentionality: The use of discourse in early child language. In D. R. Olson (Ed.), *The social foundations of language and thought.* New York: W. W. Norton & Co., 1980.

Greenfield, P. M., & Smith, J. H. *The structure of communication in early language development.* New York: Academic Press, 1976.

Grimes, J-E. *The thread of discourse.* Ithaca: Cornell University, 1972.

Halliday, M. A. K. *Learning how to mean: Explorations in the development of language.* London: Edward Arnold, 1975.

Halliday, M. A. K. Text as a semantic choice in social contexts. In T. van Dijk & J. S. Petofi (Eds.), *Grammars and descriptions,* Berlin: deGruyter, 1977.

Halliday, M. A. K., & Hasan, R. *Cohesion in English.* London: Longman, 1976.

Harste, J. C., Burke, C. L., & Woodward, V. A. *Children, their language and world: Initial encounters with print.* Final Report, Project NIE G-79-0132. Bloomington: Indiana University, 1981.

Heath, S. B. What no bedtime story means: Narrative skills at home and school. *Language in Society,* 1982, *11,* 49-79.

Holdaway, D. *The foundations of literacy.* Sydne: Ashton Scholastic, 1979.

Jusczyk, P. W., & Thompson, E. Perception of a phonetic contrast in multisyllabic utterances by 2-month-old infants. *Perception and Psychophysics,* 1978, *23,* 105-109.

Karmiloff-Smith, A. *A functional approach to child language: A study of determiners and reference.* Cambridge: Cambridge University Press, 1979.

Keenan, E. O. Making it last: Repetition in children's discourse. In S. M. Ervin-Tripp & C. Mitchell-Kernan (Eds.), *Child discourse.* New York: Academic Press, 1977.

Kinsbourne, M. Language laterilization and developmental disorders. In C. L. Ludlow & M. E. Doran-Quine (Eds.), *The neurological bases of language disorders in children: Methods and directions for research.* NINCDS Monograph No. 22. NIH Publication No. 79-440, 1979.

Kirk, U. (Ed.), *Neuropsychology of language, reading, and spelling.* New York: Academic Press, 1983.

Krashen, S. Lateralization, language learning, and the critical period: Some new evidence. *Language learning,* 1973, *23,* 63-74.

Kutas, M., & Hillyard, S. Reading between the lines: Event-related brain potentials during natural sentence processing. *Brain and Language,* 1980, *11,* 354-373.

Kutas, M., & Hillyard, S. A. The lateral distribution of event-related potentials during sentence processing. *Neuropsychologia, 20,* 1982, 579-590.

Lamendella, J. T. Relations between the ontogency and phylogeny of language: A neorecapitulationist view. *Annuals of the New York Academy of Science,* 1976, *280,* 396-412.

Lassen, N. A., Ingvar, D. H., & Skinhoj, E. Brain function and blood flow. *Scientific American,* 1978, *239,* 62-71.

Lecours, A. R. Mylogentic correlates of the development of speech and language. In E. H. Lenneberg and E. Lenneberg (Eds.), *Foundations of language development: A multidisciplinary approach,* Vol. I. New York: Academic Press, 1975.

Lennenberg, E. H. *Biological foundations of language.* New York: John Wiley, 1967.

Mandler, J. M., & Johnson, N. S. Remembrance of things past; Story structure and recall. *Cognitive Psychology,* 1977, *9,* 111-151.

Marshall, J. C. On the biology of language acquisition. In D. Caplan (Ed.) *Biological studies of mental processes.* Cambridge: The MIT Press, 1980.

Meyer, B. J. *The organization of prose and its effects on memory.* New York: American Elsevier, 1975.

Molfese, D. Neural mechanisms underlying the processing of speech information in infants and adults: Suggestions of differences in development and structure from electro-physiological research. In. U. Kirk (Ed.), *Neuropsychology of language, Reading and Spelling.* New York: Academic Press, 1983.

Molfese, D. L., & Molfese, V. J. Hemisphere and stimulus differences as reflected in the cortical responses of newborn infants to speech stimuli. *Developmental Psychology,* 1979, *15,* 505-511.

Morgan, J. L., & Green, G. M. Pragmatics and reading comprehension. In R. J. Spiro, B. C. Bruce, & W. F. Brewer. *Theoretical issues in reading comprehension: Perspectives from cognitive psychology, linguistics, artificial intelligence, and education.* Hillsdale, N. J.: Lawrence Erlbaum Associates, 1981.

Naremore, R. Studying children's language behavior: Proposing a new focus. In C. L. Ludlow & M. E. Doran-Quine (Eds.), *The neurological bases of language disorders in children: Methods and directions for research.* NINCDS Monograph No. 22. NH Publication No. 79-440, 1979.

Nelson, K. Structure and strategy in learning to talk. *Monographs of the Society for Research in Child Language,* 1973, *38,* (1-2, Serial No. 149).

Ojemann, G. A. Comments. *Neurosurgery,* 1977, *1,* 14-15.

Ojemann, G. A. Interrelationships in the brain organization of language-related behaviors: Evidence from electrical stimulation mapping. In U. Kirk (Ed.) *Neuropsychology of language, reading, and spelling.* New York: Academic Press, 1983.

Olson, D. R. From utterance to text: The bias of language in speech and writing. *Harvard Educational Review,* 1977, *47* (3), 257-281.

Orne, M. T., & Paskewitz, D. A. Adversive situational effects on alpha feedback training. *Science,* 1974, *186,* 458-460.

Orne, M., & Wilson, S. Alpha, biofeedback and arousal/activation. In J. Beatly & H. Legewie (Eds.), *Biofeedback and behavior.* New York: Plenum Press, 1977.

Penfield, W., & Roberts, L. *Speech and brain mechanisms.* New York: Atheneum, 1976.

Piaget, J. *The language and thought of the child.* London: Routledge and Kegan Paul, 1926.

Pribram, K. H. Language in a socio-biological frame. *Annuals of the New York Academy of Science*, 1976, *280*, 798-809.

Puccetti, R. The case for mental duality: Evidence from split-brain data and other considerations (with open commentary). *The Behavioral and Brain Sciences*, 1981, *4*, 93-123.

Risberg, J. Regional cerebral blood flow measures by 133-xe-inhalation methodology and applications in neuropsychology and psychiatry. *Brain and Language*, 1980, *9*, 19-34.

Risberg, J., Halsey, J. H., Wills, E. L., & Wilson, E. M. Hemispheric specialization in normal man studied by bilateral measurements of the regional cerebral blood flow: A study with the 133-xe-inhalation technique. *Brain*, 1975, *98*, 511-524.

Rosch, E. H. On the internal structure of perceptual and semantic categories. In T. E. Moore (Ed.), *Cognitive development and the acquisition of language*. New York: Academic Press, 1973.

Rose, D. Some functional correlates of the maturation of neural systems. In D. Caplan (Ed.), *Biological studies of mental processes*. Cambridge, The MIT Press, 1980.

Rumelhart, D. E. Understanding and summarizing brief stories. In D. LaBerge & S. J. Samuels (Eds.), *Basic processes in reading: Perception and comprehension*. Hillsdale, N. J.: Lawrence Erlbaum, 1977.

Satz, P. Cerebral dominance and reading disability: An old problem revisited. In R. Knights & D. J. Bakker (Eds.), *The Neuropsychology of learning disorders: Theoretical approaches*. Baltimore: University Park Press, 1975.

Schneider, G. E. Is it really better to have your brain lesion early? A revision of the "Kennard Principle." *Neuropsychologia*, 1979, *17*, 557-583.

Segalowitz, S. J. *Two sides of the brain: Brain lateralization explored*. Englewood Cliffs, N. J.: Prentice-Hall, 1983.

Serbin, L. A. Sex-differentiated free play behavior: Effects of teacher modeling, location, and gender. *Developmental Psychology*, 1981, *17*, 640-646.

Shields, M. M. The child as psychologist: Construing the social world. In A. Lock (Ed.), *Action, gesture and symbol: The emergence of language*. New York: Academic Press, 1978.

Sidman, R. L., & Rakic, P. Neural migration, with special reference to developing human brain: A review. *Brain Research*, 1973, *62*, 1-35.

Smith, F. *Understanding reading*. 3rd edition. New York: Holt, Rinehart and Winston, 1982a.

Smith, F. *Writing and the writer*. New York: Holt, Rinehart and Winston, 1982b.

Snow, C. Mothers' speech to children learning language. *Child Language*, 1972, *43*, 549-565.

Snow, C. E. Literacy and language: Relationships during the preschool years. *Harvard Educational Review*, 1983, *53*, 165-189.

Spiro, R. J., Bruce, B. C., & Brewer, W. F. (Eds.). *Theoretical issues in reading comprehension: Perspectives from cognitive psychology, linguistics, artificial intelligence, and education*. Hillsdale, N. J.: Lawrence Erlbaum Associates, 1981.

Springer, S. P., & Deutsch, G. *Left brain, right brain*. San Francisco: W. H. Freeman & Co., 1981.

Taylor, D. *Family literacy: Young children learning to read and write*. Exeter: New Hampshire: Heinemann Educational Books, 1983.

Thoman, E. B. CNS dysfunction and nonverbal communication between mother and infant. In C. L. Ludlow & M. E. Doran-Quine (Eds.), *The neurological bases of language disorders in children: methods and direction for research*. NINCDS Monograph No. 22. NIH Publication No. 79-440, 1979.

Trevarthan, C. Instincts for human understanding and for cultural cooperation: Their development in infancy. In M. vonCranach, K. Foppa, W. Lepenies, & D. Ploog, *Human ethology: Claims and limits of a new discipline*. Cambridge: Cambridge University Press, 1979.

Trevarthan, C. The foundations of intersubjectivity: Development of interpersonal and co-operative understanding in infants. In D. R. Olson (Ed.), *The social foundations of language and thought.* New York: W. W. Norton & Co., 1980.

Trevarthan, C. Development of the cerebral mechanisms for language. In U. Kirk (Ed.), *Neuropsychology of language, reading, and spelling.* New York: Academic Press, 1983.

Trevarthan, C., & Hubley, P. Secondary intersubjectivity: Confidence, confiding and acts of meaning in the first year. In A. Lock (Ed.), *Action, gesture and symbol: The emergence of language.* New York: Academic Press, 1978.

Wada, J. Prelanguage and fundamental asymmetry of the infant brain. *Annals of the New York Academy of Science,* 1977, *299,* 354, 370-379.

Wells, G. Variation in child language. In P. Fletcher & M. Garman (Eds.), *Language acquisition.* Cambridge: Cambridge University Press, 1979.

Wells, G. *Learning through interaction: The study of language development.* Cambridge: Cambridge University Press, 1981.

Whitaker, H. A., & Ojemann, G. A. Lateralization of higher cortical functions: A critique. *Annals of the New York Academy of Science,* 1977, *299,* 459-473.

Whitaker, H. A., & Selnes, O. A. Anatomic variations in the cortex: Individual differences and the problem of the localization of language functions. *Annals of the New York Academy of Sciences,* 1976, *280,* 844-854.

Witelson, S. F. Anatomical asymmetry in the temporal lobes: Its documentation, phylogenesis, and relationship to functional asymmetry. *Annals of the New York Academy of Sciences,* 1977, *299,* 328-354.

Witelson, S. F., & Pallie, W. Left hemisphere specialization for language in the newborn: Neuroanatomical evidence of asymmetry. *Brain,* 1973, *96,* 641-646.

Woods, B. T. Observations on the neurological basis for initial language acquisition. In D. Caplan (Ed.), *Biological studies of mental processes.* Cambridge: The MIT Press, 1980.

Yakovlev, P. I., & Lecours, A. R. The myelogenetic cycles of regional maturation of the brain. In Minkowski (Ed.), *Regional development of the brain in early life.* Oxford: Blackwell, 1967.

Zaidel, E. Auditory language comprehension in the right hemisphere following cerebral commissurotomy and hemispherectomy: A comparison with child language and aphasia. In A. Caramazza & E. B. Zurif (Eds.). *Language acquisition and language breakdown: Parallels and divergencies.* Baltimore: John Hopkins University Press, 1978.

Zaidel, E. The split and half brains as models of congenital language disability. In C. L. Ludlow & Doran-Quine (Eds.), *The neurological bases of language disorders in children: Methods and directions for research. NINCDS Monograph No. 22,* NIH Publication No. 79-440, 1979.

Memory Development

William V. Fabricius, MS
Henry M. Wellman, PhD

ABSTRACT. Memory development after the preschool years largely involves the acquisition of strategies for using one's memory rather than structural changes in the brain. This article reviews recent memory development research and four general principles of strategy development: (a) strategy acquisition occurs throughout the school years; (b) younger children can be trained to use strategies which are spontaneously used by older children; (c) training can result in dramatic improvements in memory performance; and, (d) children often fail to maintain and generalize trained strategies. Training needs to address children's knowledge and beliefs about memory—their metamemory—in order to achieve longer term benefits. Educational applications involve (a) determining which is the appropriate strategy to train, (b) training at the appropriate level, and (c) adapting individualized training programs to the classroom.

The basic fact of memory development is that if you observe younger and older children on just about any task which a layman would reasonably call a memory task, the younger children remember less than the older ones. This is true of tasks such as remembering numbers, words, items on a shopping list, directions on how to do a task, or foreign vocabulary. Now, in this article, titled "Memory Development," within this journal issue, titled "A Child's Brain," you might expect to read about how the anatomical and neurological growth of the brain affords and determines the development of memory. However, we will *not* be talking about the brain in that fashion. In an analogy to the now common com-

William V. Fabricius is a doctoral candidate in Developmental Psychology and Henry M. Wellman is with the Department of Psychology, The University of Michigan, Ann Arbor, MI 48109.

Preparation of this article was supported in part by a Spencer Fellowship from the National Academy of Education to the second author. Requests for reprints should be sent to the authors at the Center for Human Growth and Development, 300 North Ingalls Building, Ann Arbor, MI 48109.

puter, we will not focus on the brain's hardware (the neuroanatomy of the brain), but on the brain's software, that is, on how the brain is used in order to remember things. This, too, is brain development, but it is brain development as viewed by the cognitive psychologist rather than the biologist. The topics we will consider, then, include the strategies that children bring to bear in order to use their brains to store and retrieve information (their memory), as well as the knowledge they accumulate about their own memory (their metamemory) which helps them to devise and employ memory strategies.

Memory strategies are those things a person might do to aid his memory: things like rehearsing a phone number again and again, organizing a list into categories (nouns versus verbs for foreign vocabulary acquisition), or writing things down (shopping lists). As it turns out, focusing on strategies rather than on brain biology and neurology is particularly appropriate when discussing memory development. This is so because in the age range we focus on, the child from age 3 to adulthood, it is strategy development that accounts for most of memory development. That is, the memory differences described above are due in large part to how children of different ages use their brains, rather than to fundamental differences in their brains themselves. Resorting to the computer metaphor once again, it is not that older children have acquired radically better memory machines, but that they have become more strategic, and more knowledgeable as operators of the same machine.

TWO EXAMPLES OF MEMORY TASKS AND PERFORMANCE

To begin with, consider two children engaged in two different memory tasks. The first child, Janet, is a kindergartener, and she has left her classroom temporarily to join a pair of memory researchers. One of the experimenters shows her a page of pictures and explains that he will point to a few of the pictures, one at a time and in a certain order. She is then to close her eyes for a short while (about 15 seconds) after which all the pictures will be presented rearranged on a new page, and she must try to point out those pictures in the same order. While her eyes are closed, the other experimenter secretly watches her lips to see whether she appears to be rehearsing the sequence of picture names to herself.

The second child, Eric, is a fifth grader who has received a study assignment from his teacher. He is to read a chapter from his history book in preparation for a test in a few days. In addition, his teacher wants him to write a summary of the chapter; this should motivate him to read carefully and it will serve as a subsequent study aid.

These two examples present very different pictures in a number of respects. The differences between kindergarteners and fifth graders, even considering only performance in academic tasks, is very great. Further, the tasks are different. The first involves short-term, rote recall of a few unconnected, arbitrary items (in short, a laboratory test), and the second involves learning much more complex material for a longer period of time (the quintessential classroom task). And finally, the activities that the adults are interested in observing in the children, the strategies that might enhance memory in each case, range from simple repetition or rehearsal of individual items to sophisticated identification and summarization of the key ideas from a text.

There are, nevertheless, important similarities between the two situations, similarities that become apparent when we look at the performance of our initial children and of children a few years older in each case. Janet, the kindergartener, is almost certain to sit passively while her eyes are closed, and give no indication that she is rehearsing the pictures. A second grader, however, is likely to show some signs of rehearsal, especially if the task is repeated a number of times. Only about 25% of second graders will appear as passive as the typical kindergartener, and yet, only about 25% will consistently and clearly rehearse throughout the experiment. The rest will be notably inconsistent, appearing to rehearse on some trials but not on others. The frequency of rehearsal continues to increase through fifth grade.

In regard to the studying task, the fifth grader is likely to produce a summary of the history chapter in which relatively trivial or redundant points from the chapter have been deleted, while more important points have been copied more or less verbatim. Seventh graders, and to a greater extent tenth graders, are more likely to substitute a superordinate term for a list of exemplars, and to look for topic sentences that have been supplied by the author to include in their summaries. However, when it comes to inventing a topic sentence where one is needed, that is, expressing the implicit idea of a paragraph or paragraphs in one's own words, which is the essence of summarization, then tenth graders are likely to do this only about a third of the time, while even college students are likely to do it only about half of the time when it is appropriate. The first similarity then that one sees between these two divergent examples, when looking at changes in performance over time, is that the proportion of strategy users in each case increases relatively slowly over a number of years. In fact, research on memory development over the past 15 years has yielded a number of general principles about the development of cognitive strategies which we will consider in detail.

GENERAL PRINCIPLES OF STRATEGY DEVELOPMENT

The principles we will discuss emerged from a large and diverse body of research. Research on the development of memory strategies began with, and in some quarters continues to investigate, three main types of strategies: (a) *rehearsal,* (b) *organization or categorization,* and (c) *elaboration or imagery.* This is partly because these strategies, at least in their simpler forms, can be observed and induced in younger children, although the more complex forms continue to develop into adulthood.

For example, rehearsal in the early grade school years typically involves rote repetition of single items (Ornstein & Naus, 1978). Later, increasingly large sets of items are rehearsed in what is usually called *cumulative rehearsal* (Belmont & Butterfield, 1971). Later in grade school and high school, children refine their cumulative rehearsal strategies by planning the acquisition and retrieval components of these strategies. A study by Butterfield, Wambold and Belmont (1973) illustrates this nicely. Subjects pressed a button to view, one at a time, each of six items arranged in a line. After they had seen all of the items, at their own pace, a seventh item (the probe) was presented which was identical to one in the original six, and the subject had to indicate which position in the line it had occupied. College students handled the task by using a strategy (dubbed a *cumulative rehearsal, fast-finish* strategy) which had two components: item acquisition and retrieval. The acquisition part involved viewing the first three items and then pausing to rehearse them as a set a few times, followed by quickly viewing the last three items without rehearsal. The retrieval component involved "searching" the last three items first before their original presentation had faded from memory and, if the probe was not among them, searching the rehearsed set of items. Finally, the most sophisticated forms of rehearsal, *elaborated rehearsal*, typically appear in high school and college students. These strategies tend to reorganize the material to be rehearsed into more meaningful clusters or categories (Ornstein & Naus, 1978), thus combining with organizational strategies and resulting in longer term learning.

In addition to rehearsal, organization, and elaboration, research on memory strategies has expanded recently to include what would commonly be called *study strategies*, as implied in our example of Eric, the fifth grader and his summarization skills. Other examples of study strategies include underlining and taking notes (Brown & Smiley, 1977; 1978), outlining and mapping (Armbruster, 1979), self-questioning (Andre & Anderson, 1978; Brown, Palincsar & Armbruster, in press b), and concentrating on previously missed or difficult segments of text (Brown, Campione & Barclay, 1979; Brown, Smiley & Lawton, 1978).

First General Principle

The *first general principle* about strategy development is the one touched on above: strategy development is a long, protracted affair. There is not one age period during which children become strategic. Depending on the strategy, acquisition can occur anywhere from early grade school to college. Thus, fifth graders simultaneously appear strategic and nonstrategic, depending on whether the strategy in question is simple rehearsal or invention of topic sentences. In fact, the beginnings of strategic behavior can be observed even in preschoolers if the task used is simple and concrete enough and if strategies involve behaviors that are already well-established in the young child's repertoire (Wellman, 1977).

An example of early strategy use can be found in a study by Wellman, Ritter and Flavell (1975). Three-year-old children were shown a toy dog that was hidden, while they watched, under one of eight identical containers. The experimenter left the room for a short while, and half the children were told to "wait" with the dog while the other half were told to "remember" where the dog was. Those told to *remember* engaged in a number of behaviors apparently designed to help them recall: staring at the container which held the dog, touching it, moving it, and even nodding "yes" to that container and "no" to the others! In fact, children who showed these strategic behaviors did remember better than those who did not.

Regarding even younger children, recent work by DeLoache and Brown (1981a,b) and Wellman and Sommerville (1981) has discovered use of memory strategies in 1½ and 2-year-olds. In the DeLoache and Brown studies, for example, the child's task was to remember where a toy was hidden. The hiding places were locations in a room (behind a chair, under a pillow, etc.). Half the children played the game at their home, a familiar environment where presumably fewer strategic behaviors would be needed to remember locations, and half played the game in the laboratory, which was an unfamiliar setting that provided a more difficult task of finding an object in an unusual location. Twice as many strategic behaviors were observed in the lab, where the children needed to help themselves remember, as in the home. These memory-specific behaviors included talking about the toy or its hiding place, looking at and pointing to the hiding place, approaching the hiding location, peeking at the toy, and attempting to retrieve it early (which was prevented by the experimenter). The conclusion that children engaged in these behaviors for the purpose of remembering received further support when a control group was examined. In the control condition, a toy was placed visibly at a location and the child was made to wait before retrieving it. These children did not have to remember where the toy was (they could see it) and consequently they did not produce strategic behaviors.

Second and Third General Principles

Given that strategy development is an extremely protracted and ongoing development, the *second general principle* about that development is that for a substantial period of time before children spontaneously produce any given strategy, they can be trained to use the strategy. Training at times can be accomplished by simply asking children to produce the appropriate behavior; at other times it requires more elaborate methods. The *third general principle* is closely related to the second; when strategy production is elicited in children who do not spontaneously produce it, their performance is increased, often to a level comparable to that of older, spontaneous producers. The magnitude of this increase can be quite dramatic, sometimes 600% of an increase over initial performance (Turnure, Buium & Thurlow, 1976), or, in other terms, enough to bring retarded children up to the level of untrained college students (Butterfield et al., 1973).

The first study to investigate and demonstrate these two latter principles was done by Flavell and his coworkers (Keeney, Cannizzo & Flavell, 1967). They used the task demonstrated by Janet, the kindergartener in our first example, though this time all the children tested were first graders. Based on their performance the first day, the experimenters selected two subsets of children: those who clearly and consistently used a rehearsal strategy (the Producers), and those who did not (the Nonproducers). In a second session six weeks later, Nonproducers were given minimal training in using rehearsal; they were told to say the names of the pictures aloud when the experimenter pointed to them and then to keep whispering them over and over while their eyes were closed. The children easily understood and complied with these instructions, and on the basis of ten trials of the task under these instructions, their performance was indistinguishable from that of Producers, who continued to rehearse spontaneously.

Our second example, involving Eric, the fifth grader, can also be used to illustrate these principles and thereby demonstrate their generality across laboratory and school tasks. Day (1980) taught the summarization rules to junior college students, a population suspected of having difficulty with studying skills. In fact, prior to training, their summarizations resembled those of fifth graders; they deleted trivial and redundant points but did not use the more complex rules of superordination of exemplars of a concept, and selection and invention of topic sentences. After training, their performance especially on the more complex rules increased dramatically.

An important implication of these principles is that memory performance seems not to be so much *age-dependent* as *strategy-dependent*. In other words, much of the basic hardware of the memory system appears to be in place from a relatively early age onward, with the level of performance depending on the type of processing activity the learner performs upon the material. Recall the college level performance of young retarded children mentioned earlier. This sort of evidence has altered earlier conceptions of memory which tended to view development as the increase or growth in memory capacity or hardware with age.

The powerful effect of strategies is also illustrated by the fact that strategies can improve recall even when the child is not trying to remember. For example, in a study by Fabricius and Hagen (in press), first and second graders were presented with 12 pictures representing three common categories (such as furniture, toys, body parts), along with picture stands that would hold four pictures each. Children were told simply to "put the pictures on the stands," and most complied by sorting the pictures into categories. When they were given a surprise recall test afterward, they remembered the same amount as when they later expected a recall test to follow. The amount a child recalled was related to how completely he had sorted the pictures, whether or not he was trying to remember them.

While demonstrations of "mature" memory performances in "immature" subjects are important for the theoretical reasons mentioned above, it is important to point out that there are, not surprisingly, limits as to how effective most practical attempts at strategy training can be. There appear to be factors which affect the degree to which the strategy "takes," such as prior knowledge or familiarity with the material which the subject brings to the task, and the ability level of the subjects. For example, Day's (1980) study on summarization strategies discussed above included both average ability junior college students and those in remedial writing classes. The two groups did not differ in their use of summarization strategies prior to training. After identical training, both groups improved their use of the superordination rule to approximately the same extent. Regarding the selection and invention rules, both groups again improved but the average ability students improved significantly more than the poor writers. This divergent pattern was even more evident when a group of more severely learning impaired students, those taking both remedial reading and writing classes, was included. These latter students failed to show any improvement on the most difficult rule, invention of topic sentences. We will return to to this issue later.

Fourth General Principle

The fourth general principle sounds a pessimistic note regarding strategy training, in addition to indications of upper limits of training discussed above. Trained strategies can be irritatingly short-lived. There are two ways in which this can be the case. First, children often abandon the strategy on subsequent trials of the experiment when they are no longer told or instructed to use it. Thus, though capable of performing the strategy and benefiting from it, and in fact having just done so, they do not spontaneously use the strategy. This is usually referred to as a failure of *strategy maintenance,* and was first observed in the Keeney et al. (1967) experiment. As reported above, Nonproducers successfully rehearsed the picture names during the delay period on ten trials when they were told and reminded to whisper the names. At the end of these training trials they were told that they no longer *had* to say the names over and over, but that they could if they wanted to. On the three subsequent trials under these instructions, about 60% of the trained children showed no evidence at all of rehearsing, and less than 20% continued to rehearse consistently on those trials.

The second way in which training effect can prove ephemeral is in cases where the strategy needs not only to be maintained, but *transferred or generalized* to a new, though still appropriate task. A study by Barclay (1979) involving sixth, tenth and twelfth graders and college students provides a good example. Subjects viewed six pictures one at a time in a linear order at their own pace, and when ready had to recall them in a prescribed sequence: the last two pictures first and then the first four in order. By analyzing the time subjects took after viewing each picture, it was possible to infer how much they were rehearsing. Adults clearly used a rehearsal strategy tailored to the task, a variation of the *cumulative rehearsal, fast-finish* routine described earlier. They spent progressively longer time after each of the first four items, apparently rehearsing increasingly larger sets each time, and then quickly viewed the last two items. Thus the last two items were still fresh in memory while they were recalled first, and the initial items were learned well enough to survive a brief delay before being recalled. Few of the grade school subjects used this strategy, instead opting for a rehearsal strategy of viewing all six items and then rehearsing them as a group. When trained, however, all subjects who had not used the adult strategy were able to execute it and, importantly, were also able to spontaneously maintain use of the strategy on subsequent trials when they were no longer instructed to use it. Maintenance may have been achieved in this case because the trained strategy was a variation of a strategy subjects were already using. However, a generalization task was presented in which subjects had to view 12 pictures, representing two distinct categories of six items each. They were told ahead of time which category they would have to remember. They were to recall the pictures in the same manner (last two, first four) as before, thus making the cumulative rehearsal, fast-finish strategy still appropriate. All adults transferred the strategy to this variant of the task, but almost 80% of the sixth graders failed to show any evidence of transfer. Tenth and twelfth graders were at an intermediate level of transfer.

These four principles, (a) the almost continuous nature of strategy acquisition, (b) the trainability, and (c) effectiveness of strategies in younger children, and (d) the reversion to nonproduction after instructed use, illustrate the concept of "production deficiency" (Flavell, 1970). This refers to the fact that the development of any strategy appears to be characterized by a period during which the person simply does not produce it, although all the mechanisms for its successful execution appear to be in place. The explanation for why production deficiencies exist has proven a difficult one for developmental psychologists, and at the present time there is not widespread agreement. In the next section we will focus on one approach, the metamemory approach, to account for some of these unanswered questions about strategy development.

METAMEMORY

The term *metamemory* refers to a person's knowledge (or beliefs) about memory and how it works, knowledge which then might be used to decide when and where to use certain strategies (Flavell & Wellman, 1977). The idea is that production deficiencies might occur because the person simply does not think to use the strategy, or in other words, because the person's knowledge about memory (metamemory) does not include that particular strategic activity as a useful or relevant activity for the particular materials and task at hand. To return once again to our helpful kindergartener, perhaps she and many of her schoolmates in first and second grade were not aware that whispering the names of the pictures during the delay period would help them remember, even after they had done so in response to the experimenter's instructions. As Flavell put it in an insightful comment at the time, "There was of course no explicit feedback to the children as to the effects of rehearsal on their recall performance, and this may have been partly responsible for this rapid extinction of the verbalization strategy" (Keeney et al., 1967, pp. 961-962).

It was not until 1976 that this possibility was directly tested. Kennedy and Miller (1976) repeated the Keeney et al., procedure, except that this time half of the Nonproducers were given the following feedback after training and before the final three trials on which they were told they did not have to rehearse: "My goodness, you did so much better when you whispered those names over and over. I guess whispering helped you remember the pictures better. Right?" (Kennedy & Miller, 1976, p. 567). All the children who received this feedback continued to rehearse on the last three trials, whereas only about 10% of the trained Nonproducers without feedback did so. Since then, other studies have shown similar effects (Paris, Newman & McVey, in press; Ringle & Springer, 1980). In fact, Day's (1980) summary-writing training study included this type of feedback, and those average ability junior college students who responded to initial training continued to show improvement in classroom assignments from their teachers several weeks later, an impressive demonstration of maintenance and generalization.

Evidence from studies such as these can be related to other evidence we have about strategy training and acquisition to suggest both a theoretical perspective and a framework for educational applications. We know first of all that normal children come to acquire all of the strategies investigated by developmental psychologists (plus many more!) on their own without explicit instruction. By themselves, they come to strategies which are optimal for certain frequently seen tasks and materials, and in addition can rather quickly compile specialized routines (such as cumulative rehearsal fast-finish strategies) adapted to even novel, arbitrary tasks. Furthermore, it appears that strategy acquisition may be more accurately described as strategy replacement (Brown, Bransford, Ferrara & Compione, in press a). That is, it is seldom the case that the child is doing nothing before coming to apply a strategy such as rehearsal or categorization. Recall the simple but strategic memory efforts of even pre-school children reviewed earlier. Rather, more efficient strategies come to replace less efficient ones. For example, in the Fabricius and Hagen (in press) study, while not all children knew that categorization had improved their recall, nevertheless very few failed to mention something they had done ("looked at the pictures," "said them," "studied them," etc.) to help themselves remember. These considerations suggest that the child may be engaged in some type of hypothesis generation and testing process regarding the effectiveness of various memory strategies. As we have seen, there are periods in development when children will produce a strategy in some trials of an experiment (or in some situations in "real life") and not in others. Factors such as the child's discovery that recall varies depending on whether or not she has produced the strategy, and/or the child's insight into possible mechanisms by which the strategy works (such as categorization working by means of associations among items) may be important for the child's development of hypotheses about memory.

Wellman and his colleagues (Fabricius & Hagen, in press; Fabricius & Wellman, 1983; Wellman, 1982, in press) have recently characterized the child's developing metamemory as a naive "theory of mind." According to this view, the child develops a more and more interrelated system of beliefs about what types of factors affect memory, their relative effects depending on the task or situation, how they interact with the child's abilities and prior knowledge, and their relative costs (in terms of effort) and benefits. This view of metamemory appears to map well onto much of what we know about strategy development, and suggests that training and intervention efforts should consider the child's view of the trained strategy. This means assuring that the child sees the trained strategy not only useful but as more useful than his or her previous efforts, and understands how and why it is applicable for a certain range of tasks. Other issues involved in the educational applications of strategy training are discussed below.

EDUCATIONAL APPLICATIONS

The view of memory development presented above has many obvious educational implications since it shows the younger child to be an able but "unschooled" rememberer. The child needs to learn various memory and study strategies. However, the training of strategies involves teaching students how to learn rather than teaching them course content. At the end of the year, however, it is course content for which teachers are held accountable. For this reason learning skills or strategies tend not to be taught explicitly in the schools (Brown et al., in press a). Yet it is clearly the case that many students have not acquired effective study skills on their own initiative.

The *first* issue in teaching strategies is to know which strategies are actually effective for which tasks. The results of controlled laboratory experiments are most useful here. Unfortunately, at the present more is known about strategies that work for rote-type learning or memory tasks than for comprehension-based learning from texts. Of course rote memorization strategies are themselves important (Wagner, in press) since many of the school tasks of the younger child require memorizing sets of information: vocabulary items, spelling, addition facts. Even for tasks such as these it is not always easy or straightforward to determine which strategy is optimal and thus should be taught. For example, Pressley (reviewed in Pressley, Levin, & Bryant, 1983) has investigated a key-word method for vocabulary learning. The key-word method is an elaboration strategy in which, for example, the meaning of *carlin*—an old woman—is learned by forming an image of an old woman getting into, or driving, a car. The key word method has been tested against a variety of semantic or memory-based strategies which are typically recommended by reading theorists (Johnson & Pearson, 1978). Semantic strategies include providing words that are meaningfully related to the vocabulary items, providing more specific definitions, including the words in sentences, and providing pictures representing the meanings of the words. All of these seem like reasonable educational approaches. Yet Pressley has found that the key-word method is superior to such semantic strategies. Furthermore, students trained to use the semantic strategies did no better than students who were given no strategy training at all!

If research is necessary to determine which strategies to teach for simpler memorization tasks, then this is even more true for comprehension and recall of written matter. In fact, the more complex the strategy and learning situation, the less useful are naive, intuitive theories about what procedures lead to better learning. An illustration of the need to investigate the effectiveness of strategies before they are taught can be found in Day's (1980) study of summarization skills. She employed a control condition in which one group of junior college students received training similar to traditional summary writing instructions: be economical with words, include all the main ideas, etc. Her treatment groups received instruction in the five rules of deletion or trivia and redundancy, superordination, and selection and invention of topic sentences. These rules had been uncovered in previous research (Brown & Day, in press), where it was also learned that they formed a hierar-

chy of increasing difficulty. The traditional writing instructions
proved inferior to the research-derived strategies.

A *second issue* involves the level at which strategy instruction
should be aimed. Brown et al. (in press a) have distinguished between *specific skills,* such as specific types of rehearsal, elaboration or summary-writing, and *general skills,* which include selecting, sequencing, and coordinating specific skills. For example,
Butterfield et al. (1973) encountered this problem when training
the cumulative rehearsal, fast-finish strategy discussed earlier. After a number of attempts, they discovered that effective training required (a) training the acquisition strategy of rehearsing the first
items and quickly viewing the last, (b) training the retrieval strategy of searching the last items in memory first, and finally (c) *explicitly* training the sequence and coordination of the two. Similarly, Day (1980) in her study found that explicit training
involving the management of the five summarization rules was necessary in some cases. Specifically, for the most complex summarization rule, invention of topic sentences, some average junior
college students needed general-level as well as specific-level
training in order to succeed well, whereas for the less complex
rules specific-level training alone was sufficient. It should be noted
that the complexity of any strategy is a function not only of the
strategy, but also of the learner's ability. When training is ineffec-
tive at the specific level, it may mean that the strategy needs to be
broken down into its component processes and training directed at
their step-by-step coordination. These considerations mean that
students who appear to have reached their upper limits in terms of
strategy training may only need additional training at a more general level.

Finally, a *third* and even more problematic issue involves how
strategy training can be practically accomplished at a group level
in the classroom. This issue, and others, are discussed by Peterson
and Swing (1983). Again, as strategy complexity increases, this
becomes more of an issue. As an example, Brown et al. (in press
b) conducted what is perhaps the most "ecologically valid" strategy training attempted to date. The training was done individually
with seventh graders who had severe comprehension problems:

> Over many sessions, the tutor and the child engaged in an
> interactive learning game that involved taking turns in lead-
> ing a dialogue concerning each segment of text. Both the tu-

tor and the child would read a text segment, and then the dialogue leader would paraphrase the main idea, question any ambiguities, predict the possible questions that might be asked about that segment and hypothesize about the content of the remaining passage segments. The dialogue leader would then ask the other a question on the segment. In the next segment, the roles were reversed. (Brown et al., in press a, p. 134-135.)

The design of the training was based on theory and empirical findings. Further, the students were told how and why the techniques were useful, were given feedback about effectiveness, and were told they should use them any time they studied. This labor-intensive training paid off: recall and comprehension improved 500-600% on passages students read *independently* both in the lab *and* in the classroom. Even in other, more modest training studies the training is usually individually administered. Thus, what is needed are both workable classroom techniques and materials which incorporate the necessary aspects of training, and well-designed research to evaluate the effects of group-based training. As the strategic components of memory and learning are better understood, it appears more and more that we can devise the technology for their improvement. Yet the task of translating that technology into efficient educational practice is one in which educators and psychologists will have to join forces.

REFERENCES

Andre, M. D. A., & Anderson, T. H. The development and evaluation of a self-questioning study technique. *Reading Research Quarterly,* 1978/1979, *14,* 605-623.

Armbruster, B. B. *An investigation of the effectiveness of "mapping" text as a study strategy for middle school students.* Unpublished doctoral dissertation, University of Illinois, 1979.

Barclay, C. R. The executive control of mnemonic activity. *Journal of Experimental Child Psychology,* 1979, *27,* 262-276.

Belmont, J. M., & Butterfield, E. C. Learning strategies as determinants of memory deficiencies. *Cognitive Psychology,* 1971, *2,* 411-420.

Brown, A. L., Bransford, J. D., Ferrara, R. A., & Campione, J. C. Learning, Remembering, and Understanding. In J. H. Flavell and E. M. Markman (Eds.), *Carmichael's Manual of Child Psychology* (Vol. 1). New York: Wiley, in press (a).

Brown, A. L., Campione, J. C., & Barclay, C. R. Training self-checking routines for estimating test readiness: Generalizations from list learning to prose recall. *Child Development,* 1979, *50,* 501-512.

Brown, A. L., & Day, J. D. Macrorules for summarizing texts: The development of expertise. *Journal of Verbal Learning and Verbal Behavior,* in press.

Brown, A. L., Palincsar, A. S., & Armbruster, B. B. Inducing comprehension-fostering activities in interactive learning situations. In H. Mandl, N. Stein, & T. Trabasso (Eds.), *Learning from texts.* Hillsdale, N.J.: Erlbaum, in press (b).

Brown, A. L., & Smiley, S. S. Rating the importance of structural units of prose passages: A problem of metacognitive development. *Child Development,* 1977, *48,* 1-8.

Brown, A. L., & Smiley, S. S. The development of strategies for studying texts. *Child Development,* 1978, *49,* 1076-1088.

Brown, A. L., Smiley, S. S., & Lawton, S. Q. C. The effects of experience on the selection of suitable retrieval cues for studying texts. *Child Development,* 1978, *49,* 829-835.

Butterfield, E. C., Wambold, C., & Belmont, J. M. On the theory and practice of improving short-term memory. *American Journal of Mental Deficiency,* 1973, *77,* 654-669.

Day, J. D. *Training summarization skills: A comparison of teaching methods.* Unpublished doctoral dissertation, University of Illinois, 1980.

DeLoache, J. S., & Brown, A. L. *Precursors of mnemonic strategies in very young children's memory for the location of hidden objects.* Unpublished manuscript, University of Illinois, 1981 (a).

DeLoache, J. S., & Brown, A. L. *Young children's memory for the location of objects hidden in large- and small-scale spaces.* Unpublished manuscript, University of Illinois, 1981 (b).

Fabricius, W. V., & Hagen, J. H. The use of causal attributions about recall performance to assess metamemory and predict strategic memory behavior in young children. *Developmental Psychology,* in press.

Fabricius, W. V., & Wellman, H. M. Children's understanding of retrieval cue utilization. *Developmental Psychology,* 1983, *19,* 15-21.

Flavell, J. H. Developmental studies of mediated memory. In H. W. Reese & L. P. Lipsitt (Eds.), *Advances in child development and behavior* (Vol. 5). New York: Academic Press, 1970.

Flavell, J. H., & Wellman, H. M. Metamemory. In R. V. Kail, Jr., & J. W. Hagen (Eds.), *Perspectives on the development of memory and cognition.* Hillsdale, N.J.: Erlbaum, 1977.

Johnson, D. D., & Pearson, P. D. *Teaching reading vocabulary.* New York: Holt & Co., 1978.

Keeney, T. J., Cannizzo, S. R., & Flavell, J. H. Spontaneous and induced verbal rehearsal in a recall task. *Child Development,* 1967, *38,* 953-966.

Kennedy, B. A, & Miller, D. J. Persistent use of verbal rehearsal as a function of information about its value. *Child Development,* 1976, *47,* 566-569.

Ornstein, P. A., & Naus, M. J. Rehearsal processes in children's memory. In P. A. Ornstein (Ed.), *Memory organization and structure.* Hillsdale, N.J.: Erlbaum, 1978.

Paris, S. G., Newman, R. S., & McVey, K. A. From tricks to strategies: Learning the functional significance of mnemonic actions. *Journal of Experimental Child Psychology,* 1982, *34,* 490-509.

Peterson, P. L., & Swing, S. R. Problems in classroom implementation of cognitive strategy instruction. In M. Pressley & J. R. Levin (Eds.), *Cognitive strategy research: Educational applications.* New York: Springer-Verlag, 1983.

Pressley, M., Levin, J. R., & Bryant, S. L. Memory strategy instruction during adolescence: When is explicit instruction needed? In M. Pressley and J. R. Levin (Eds.), *Cognitive strategy research: Psychological foundations.* New York: Springer-Verlag, 1983.

Ringle, B. A., & Springer, C. On knowing how well one is remembering: The persistence of strategy use during transfer. *Journal of Experimental Child Psychology,* 1980, *29,* 322-333.

Turnure, J. W., Buium, N., & Thurlow, M. L. The effectiveness of interrogatives for prompting verbal elaboration productivity in young children. *Child Development,* 1976, *47,* 851-855.

Wagner, D. A. Rediscovering "rote": Some cognitive and pedagogical preliminaries. In S.

Irvine & J. W. Berry (Eds.), *Human assessment and cultural factors*. New York: Plenum, in press.

Wellman, H. M. The early development of intentional memory behavior. *Human Development*, 1977, *20*, 86-101.

Wellman, H. M. A child's theory of mind: The development of conceptions of cognition. In S. Yussen (Ed.), *The growth of insight in the child*. New York: Academic Press, 1982.

Wellman, H. M. Metamemory revisited. In M. T. H. Chi (Ed.), *What is memory development the development of? A look after a decade*. *Human Development*, in press.

Wellman, H. M., Ritter, K., & Flavell, J. H. Deliberate memory behavior in the delayed reactions of very young children. *Developmental Psychology*, 1975, *11*, 780-787.

Wellman, H. M., & Sommerville, S. C. Quasi-naturalistic tasks in the study of cognition: The memory-related skills of toddlers. *New Directions for Child Development*, 1980, *10*, 33-48.

Cognitive Rehabilitation and the Head-Injured Child

Kevin Henry, MEd

ABSTRACT. The dynamics of head injury, particularly for children, pose a challenge for rehabilitation professionals. While a great deal of information has come to the fore in recent years elucidating the nature of brain-behavior relationships, it has focused primarily upon diagnostic considerations. Attention to the development of improved techniques of treatment is becoming increasingly widespread. Cognitive rehabilitation therapy is an emerging branch of rehabilitation attempting to address the intervention needs of traumatically head injured children. Its full consideration must encompass relevant knowns in neuropsychology, patterns of recovery of victims, its place in a growing Cognitive Science, and a functional view of cognitive processes upon which responsible treatment may be based.

INTRODUCTION

Studying children and adults who have suffered head injuries is not new in contemporary society. Levin, Benton, and Grossman (1982) have documented a rich history of intervention that stretches back over several millenia. The past several decades have seen an explosion of information relating to the needs of these victims, however. The convergence of various fields in neurology and social science have contributed to the rapid advancement of knowledge of cerebral functions and processes that are affected by trauma.

Primary leadership in the increased understanding of brain-behavior relationships and the ensuing dysfunctions that occur when a head injury has been suffered has been provided by neuropsychologists. A. R. Luria has been one such major influence, W. C. Halstead another. The work of these and many other skilled psy-

---

Kevin Henry is a cognitive rehabilitation therapist at The Rehabilitation Institute of Pittsburgh, Pittsburgh, PA 15217.

189

chologists has tended to focus attention on acquiring diagnostic expertise in the localization of brain lesions. Observing a patient's performance of specific diagnostic tasks has become the foremost area of interest in work with the head-injured.

Currently, Ralph Reitan is one such neuropsychologist who is and has been long acknowledged as an authority on brain-behavior relationships. He recently made a particularly telling remark.[1] Asked what he envisions to be the major trends forthcoming in neuropsychology, he answered with confidence that the next ten years would bring to his field, so given to sophistication in brain-behavior *diagnosis*, increased interest in the commitment to *rehabilitation*. Clearly, he was suggesting the increasing importance of the role of treatment for the head injured. He recalled that he used to be gently confronted by a neurosurgeon friend who apparently was sometimes irritatingly long on empathy. After reviewing together the nature of the cerebral insult that a mutual patient had suffered and projecting the cognitive deficiencies the patient whould likely face, Dr. Reitan was persistently queried by his friend, "Ralph, what are we going to do to help this fellow?" Dr. Reitan related that, until recently, his own irritated answer would be something to the effect that he would retrain the traumatized patient's brain back to a level of functional ability as soon as his neurosurgeon friend "starting getting his paraplegic patients to walk again." Today, apparently, he views the question differently.

Understanding and skill in the *treatment* of head injured patients is indeed beginning to catch up with the strides of diagnosis. Though they are still in relatively early stages, it is possible to delineate some of the more important considerations of these treatment efforts. The present article will discuss the development of this field of rehabilitation, particular concerns at various stages of a patient's recovery, some fundamental principles of treatment, and a way in which clinicians may think about cognition. The head injured child of school age who is capable developmentally of viewing himself as a learner will be the focus of attention.

---

[1]Comments made at "Advanced Workshop in Neuropsychological Evaluation and Interpretation," Atlantic City, June 1983.

COGNITIVE REHABILITATION THERAPY

Clinicians in rehabilitation have been grappling with the challenge posed by Dr. Reitan's friend for some time. Their collective efforts to provide the help that children who have suffered traumatic brain damage so desperately need have helped to fashion what is rapidly becoming a distinct arm of rehabilitation. This field, Cognitive Rehabilitation Therapy (CRT), is strikingly interdisciplinary in its best form. It is comprised of speech-language pathologists, occupational therapists, and special education teachers: it is heavily dependent on and tied to the skills of psychologists, social workers, and computer scientists. Accordingly, it involves the talents and skills of all these professionals in the evaluatory, treatment, and follow-up phases of comprehensive rehabilitation.

This newly forming arm of rehabilitation seems to be bursting with energetic growth. Its sensitivity to the findings of cognitive science and its eagerness to translate that burgeoning science's discoveries into functional benefits for the head injured have made it an enticingly current area of rehabilitation. Due to the rising incidences of automobile accidents, coupled with increased efficiency of life-saving techniques in acute-care hospitals, it is developing at a rapid pace. It is also attended by some controversy: the heavy investment by third party payers necessitates justification in terms of theory and convincing clinical results. And without doubt it is an expanding enterprise. The numbers of rehabilitation agencies that now offer CRT programs are on a dramatic upswing.

The National Head Injury Foundation refers to these traumatized children as a "silent epidemic," reflecting their increasing numbers and the particularly devastating problems that their resultant cognitive difficulties imply. This newly evolving arm of rehabilitation is a response to that growing epidemic. Team-based, grounded in cognitive science, and surrounded by some controversy, it is an emerging effort to take seriously the question, "What are we going to do to help these children?" Expanding the question, it asks, "How are we to assist head injured children so that their residual strengths may be maximized, their weaknesses minimized, their spontaneous recovery channeled, and their optimal independence reachieved?"

Traumatic head injury automatically implies suddenly disordered processes of perceiving, thinking, understanding, reasoning, remembering, interacting with others, and evaluating oneself. Recognizing this, cognitive rehabilitation must first come to grips with the patterns of recovery that the child who has lost these fundamental skills will exhibit.

STAGES OF RECOVERY

Rancho Los Amigos, a rehabilitation center that has provided in the past decade a pioneering spirit of education and training for professionals wanting to know more about closed head injuries, has made a lasting contribution with its outline of such stages of recovery. Distilled from front-line clinical work, their "Levels of Cognitive Functioning" (1980) have served as a very useful guideline for tracking progress in the head injured patient's path toward intellectual/linguistic restoration; they have also meshed well with the typical patterns of recovery noted by other rehabilitation agencies whose numbers of head injured patients have permitted similar observations. The "Rancho Levels" consist of eight stages of clusters of behaviors that are felt to characterize a patient's line of movement—from no response to stimulation in the worst cases, i.e., coma, to a final stage of purposeful and appropriate behavior. The progression of stages reflect the somewhat predictable-but by no means predetermined-regaining of abilities such as increased awareness, orientation, memory, social appropriateness, and independence that are gradually (or sometimes quickly) reachieved from considerably more modest and less functional levels of ability commonly resulting from head traumas.

At The Rehabilitation Institute of Pittsburgh the Head Injury Team has adapted from the Rancho Levels a similar though abbreviated conceptual framework of recovery with which to view treatment planning for the head injured child. Three stages are used, essentially reflecting the combining of the Rancho Levels 1-3, 4-6, and 7-8, and are referred to as Early, Middle, and Late Stages of Recovery. Though a foreshortened form, this framework provides in larger chunks the same important considerations necessary for responsible planning and useful intervention.

Very briefly outlined, those considerations of treatment include such as the following.

Early Stages of Recovery

These stages begin functionally at the end of coma. Environmental restructuring is essential in order to meet the child's needs. High degrees of *consistency* are required in routines, people with whom the child will work, and verbal input the child will receive. Due to gross confusion and disorientation, the child at this stage is frequently agitated, incoherent, and bizarre. The environment should therefore include as much familiarity as possible (favorite personal objects, pictures, toys, music, etc.). Though the child may be largely unresponsive, some intact perceptual and language processing skills should be assumed and controlled stimulation of this kind introduced. The tone of talk and general approach should be comforting, calming, and reassuring.

Middle Stages of Recovery

As the child becomes more capable of task-related responsiveness, systematic and hierarchical presentation of tasks becomes even more important and should be provided as the child's frustration levels permit. Generally, the progression of stimulus-response tasks are presented in order of:

1. visual-motor (sorting, matching, block design...)
2. auditory-motor (following simple directions...)
3. auditory-verbal (story comprehension tasks...).

The rules of thumb are to move from simple to complex, from concrete to abstract, from passive to active involvement of the child in increasingly more demanding levels of work. Goal-setting that is consistent with the child's rate of movement toward greater tolerance for tasks and that assures a high rate of success is needed. The levels of difficulty of work must be continually assessed to match the child's spurts of recovery. Manipulating the variables that are crucial in the quality of the child's reduced but recuperating information processing abilities is essential. The rate, amount, duration, complexity, and degree and kinds of distractions present during the performance of tasks must therefore be continually modified to both meet the child at his present level as well as to challenge his re-emerging abilities. Frequent positive feedback is crucial, not only to maximize the child's motivation, but also to help develop and improve skills of self-monitoring and self-evaluating the accuracy and quality of his own performance, teaching him to see how well he meets task goals. These meta-cognitive skills (sometimes called executive functions since they bespeak control and self-direction—being in the drivers' seat) play in an increasingly important role in further recovery and, for that matter, life-long self-organization.

Late Stages of Recovery

Treatment now can and should become more specifically related to particular areas of cognitive dysfunction. Concentrated work in areas such as language processing, judgment, and inferential reasoning should be undertaken. Work in therapy settings should now interface with real-life, functional situations in which the child will eventually find himself. For most, that will mean beginning to approximate the demands that will be included in future school placements. Included in task selections should be requirements of skill integration. It is commonplace for head injured children in these latter stages of recovery to demonstrate strong performance in tasks of single modality input-output requirements (such as discussing a story heard); it is just as commonplace for them to fall apart when presented with tasks involving cross-modal learning, or integration of several input-output channels (such as describing a picture seen).

In this phase of treatment structures of support should be gradually and systematically faded, greater levels of independence and social appropriateness prioritized as goals, and frustration tolerance built. The accent now becomes concentratedly to help the child gain insight into his particular strengths and weaknesses, and to recognize and use other internal and external assists. Specifically, the child will need to become familiar with strategies of compensation for learning with which he may compose and assist himself in future situations of confusion or cognitive difficulty. The success or failure of those strategies may be pivotal. They may be the difference between having a way to deal with a problem, or having none, and facing resultantly greater confusion and embarrassment. For the nontraumatized child, learning becomes over time a rather automatic, second nature process, rarely needing exaggerated means of effort other than traditional studying. For the head injured child, deliberate, conscious consideration of seemingly obvious steps necessary for the completion of routine tasks or the solving of simple problems may be frequently needed. It is imperative in the latter stages of treatment to try to reinstate that status of more "second-nature" styles of learning, while helping the child to habituate and internalize new strategies for learning with which he may compensate for the inevitable learning difficulties ahead.

Treatment for children in these latter stages of recovery can be tricky. Often a child at this point shows no obvious signs of having suffered perhaps only months before so devastating an experience as a head trauma. Becky, a very bright and nicely recovering twelve-year-old who was performing at grade level during the final phase of her treatment once turned in to her therapist an answer sheet on which she had been working. She had just finished an independent reading assignment requiring her to write answers to questions at the end of the story she had read in a textbook. Her paper was nicely organized (good sign); her writing was spatially intact, neat, with no spelling or worrisome perceptual errors (good signs). A quick glance at her answers showed concise but fluid written expression, complete sentences grammatically correct (very good signs). Curiously, however, for question six she had drawn what was very clearly a person on a bicycle, followed by a car, then a bus (strange signs). The drawing amidst the written answers was a conspicuous oddity. Her therapist quickly checked the teacher's manual to see what question all this was supposed to answer. Question six was, "What conclusion can you draw from this story about getting around in a crowded city?" And, the manual's answer: "In a crowded city you can often get somewhere quicker by bicycle than by car or bus." Becky had indeed *drawn* the correct conclusion (good sign, but with qualification).

PRINCIPLES OF TREATMENT

In considering the cognitive rehabilitation of head injured children, there are certain principles undergirding treatment at all stages that warrant additional comment.

The plasticity of the child's brain. Damaged neurons in the brain do not regrow at critical sites. However, given that the child's brain develops and matures as assuredly as the rest of him, it may be thought of in its youth as more "healable." It may be better able to recover from the sheering, tearing, and twisting dynamics within the skull that attend most head traumas. There is debate on the question. The less mature brain may, as some studies suggest, exhibit greater resilience to the effects of focal brain lesions. Other studies indicate that the child's brain may be more susceptible to the effects of diffuse damage. To what extent and under what conditions of injury the child's recovery may be enhanced by its youth are unclear. The ambiguity on the question, however, ought not to eclipse continuing to direct treatment efforts toward stimulating remedial cortical activity. It is reasonable to assume that certain tasks fire activity in the young brain adjacent to sites of damaged tissue, encouraging a kind of "take over" of functioning by the spared and more easily influenced neighboring brain regions. The principle is an important one in the justification of intervention and rehabilitative programming.

The element of new learning. The head injured child is disadvantaged by his paucity of old learning and immensity of new learning ahead. A head injury, almost by definition, will more significantly impair the acquisition of new information than the relearning of old information. For the child, life is primarily future. Age, developmental maturity, and the strength of pretraumatic learning become important issues. The more central issue for the therapist, however, becomes discerning how the head injured child now learns, of finding and teaching for each patient the most effective methods of acquiring, interpreting, storing, recalling, and using *new* information.

Advances in Cognitive Science. More stuff is coming out than ever before on the nature of brain-behavior relationships and human information processing. Therapists and teachers immediately benefit, to the extent they are willing to keep up; their goal-setting, treatment, and follow-up efforts have on their side some of the best minds around. Recent research in the neurosciences on left-right hemispheric functions as well as the more clinically important findings on such pragmatic topics as attention and memory have been downright exciting. The bursting upon the scene of computer science and its work in artificial intelligence have and will be monumental. There is an almost mysterious justice and beauty in the confluence of those incisive minds of science in various ways touching the shattered worlds of the head injured. The cognitive rehabilitation therapist straddles the point of contact and helps make the exchange meaningful, making the science work for the patient and in turn humanizing and enlarging the science. It's not a bad place to be, but staying up to date with what the science has to offer becomes imperative.

The multi-dimensionality of cognition. Cognition is a process, not an entity, more a "how" than a "what." Understanding the dynamic nature of myriad simultaneous or rapidly sequential operations that are cognition can be perplexing. Sorting out which process(es) may be hindering the child's learning of a given task is critical. The therapist who must decide if a child's difficulty with, say, following verbal directions may ask whether the problem is attention or memory, difficulty with receptive language, a lack of strategies for oganizing information, emotional dysfunctions, or perhaps an inadequately processed environment. The list of questions can go on because the untangling of processes brought to bear in the child's performance of a task is a constant in treatment. It becomes all the more crucial, therefore, for the therapist to become experienced in task-analysis. Developing skill in sorting out those complex processes and perceiving their roles in the execution of tasks selected for treatment are vital.

Compensatory strategies as the apex of treatment. The foregoing principles all funnel to this. The bottom line that the responsible cognitive therapist aches to know is how this head injured child now learns. To understand this is to know how to select, plan for, and begin to teach compensatory strategies. The success of treatment, broadly considered, may well hinge in the end on how well those compensatory strategies have been selected and taught, because they largely determine how independent the child becomes in his own new learning.

Three components are essential in training for their use:

1. Selecting strategies that are right, that fit the child's neuro-psychological status of spared brain functions and abilities.
2. Teaching the child to discriminate the occasions and need for their implementation, helping him to experience success with their use.
3. Habituating their use, maximizing their internalization, and generalizing their use to functional settings other than those of therapy. This demands the involvement and training as well of parents, teachers, and significant others in the child's life.

The kinds of compensatory strategies to be taught are as varied as the child's strengths. A complete listing here is, as they say, beyond the scope of the present article, but a few examples are offered in the following section.

A FRAMEWORK FOR CONCEPTUALIZING COGNITION

A fundamental way to understand cognition is needed if its disorders are to be recognized and responsibly treated. Researchers have generated various models which tend differentially to emphasize processing systems, learning procedures, and anatomical structures, and their insights have been valuable. The position of this article, however, is that theory exclusivity should be avoided and an eclectic and flexible viewpoint maintained. For professionals involved in treatment, the essential question is not so much, "Which theory is best?" as, "Which model allows me to know what basic operations to look for, observe this child's strengths and deficits, and set legitimate, realistic goals?" The keynote really is, "What is the most *functional* way to think about cognition?"

The following is therefore offered, not as an ideal conceptualization, but as one way to view cognition functionally. Included are related questions the clinician frequently asks, and some strategies that may be considered in seeking to teach a child a means of compensation for his deficits.

1. *Attention*:

- How well does the child pay attention?
- For how long?
- Can he selectively attend, screening out unimportant competing stimuli during the presentation or performance of a task?
- Is his concentration adequate, or does it wane or become easily diverted?
- Can he shift attention between persons, events, topics, etc.

Strategies:

- Teach use of habitual self-instruction such as, "Am I paying attention? Do I need to look? To listen?"

2. *Orientation*:

- Is the child aware of and oreinted to persons, times, routines?
- Is he aware of his own condition, the reasons for and goals of treatment?

Strategies:

- Teach the child to refer to written or pictured cues (a miniature guide with vital personal information and photos).
- Teach the child to use deliberate and methodical scanning of the immediate environment for needed cues.

3. *Perceptual Processing*:

- Are there modality-specific dysfunctions?
- In either visual or auditory realms, what are the child's abilities of closure, discrimination, and figure ground?
- Are there problems of visual field neglect?
- Could deficiencies in perception be affecting higher level skills I'm trying to teach?

Strategies:

- Teach methodical means of scanning a visual field, steps to follow in looking such as, "Start in the upper left and go right..."
- Teach use of the best angle of vision for capturing optimal visual fields, or deliberate self-instruction such as "Look to the left" if field neglect is a problem.

4. *Language Processing*:

- For material the child either hears or reads, what is his level of ability for

  — vocabulary mastery?
  — the rate at which information comes?
  — the amount with which he can deal?
  — the length of time he can profitably work?
  — the distractions he can tolerate?
  — the complexity/distraction levels he can handle?

- Can the child distill main ideas from extented amounts of talk?
- Does he understand idiomatic language, or does he tend to be literal-minded (remember Becky's drawing her conclusions?)?
- Is the child impaired in the contextual aspects of language (the pragmatics of speech acts and discourses)?

Strategies:

- Teach the child to use techniques of input control, such as asking a speaker to slow down, to restate, or to clarify directions and messages.
- Teach overt/covert summarizing skills, the child perhaps being trained to ask, "Let me see if I understand you. Did you say..."
- Teach the child to internalize a visual framework (a simple chart or diagram) for organizing thematic information that would include the salient details of who, what, where, when, why, how.

5. *Expressive Language:*

- Does the child initiate conversations appropriately?
- Does he elaborate meaningfully on themes, or add irrelevant information, or become otherwise disorganized?
- Does he perseverate or confabulate?
- Does he have trouble retrieving words he wishes to use in conversations?

Strategies:

- Teach habitual self-instruction such as, "What's my main point?" or, "Am I being clear?"
- Teach deliberate scanning of listener's facial expressions for cues indicating a need to clarify his talk.
- Teach the child to actively query a listener, "Am I being clear?"
- For word retrieval difficulties, teach the child to generate categories, attributes, or associations of the word sought, or perhaps to gesture or even draw the concept if possible.

6. *Problem-Solving*:

- Does the child recognize problem situations?
- Is he cognizant of goals that problems imply?
- Does he recognize a need for acquiring relevant information?
- Can he ask for needed information in appropriate ways?
- Can he discriminate relevant from irrelevant information?
- Does he remain mindful of goals when trying to generate solutions to problems, or become overinvolved in details?
- Do time pressures significantly impair his clarity of thought or quality of output?
- Are fatigue thresholds too quickly overreached?
- Does he become easily frustrated, confused, or rigid in thinking?
- Is he easily overloaded by even helpful and relevant input from others?
- Is he realistic in generating solutions?
- Can he appropriately choose among various solutions?
- Can he foresee new problems created by some solutions?
- Can he make a reasonable plan of action?
- Can he carry-through on such a plan?

Strategies:

- Teach and habituate consideration of the critical steps of problem-solving implied above.
- Teach child to self-instruct with critical questions such as, "What will happen if I...?", or, "What *else* can I do to solve this problem?" or, "Can someone else help me on this?"

7. *Reasoning*:

- Does the child show ability to reason thematically?
- Can he reason analogically (Emergent around 7 years)?
- Is he unduly concrete in reasoning, or does he make age-appropriate inferences?
- Does he seem to be stimulus-bound, or can he discern similarities and differences between people, objects, ideas, and events?

Strategies:

- Teach and habituate comparisons based on semantic feature analyses of categories, actions, uses, locations, properties/attributes, and strong associations (through discussions, for example, of the similarities and differences between dogs and cats, ice cream and cake, Smurfs and Flintstones, Pac Man and Donkey Kong...).

8. *Memory:*

- Are memory problems specific for recalling personal events or for organized aspects of expected conceptual knowledge (episodic vs. semantic memory)?
- Is the difficulty for recently given information, or long term recall, or both?
- Is the difficulty more with encoding (input), storage, or retrieval of information?
- Is the problem more of a content-specific or modality-specific nature?
- Are there significant discrepancies between levels of retention for information that is:

    —visual vs. verbal?
    —intentional vs. incidental?
    —past vs. things to be done in the future?
    —novel vs. familiar
    —structured vs. unstructured

- Does the child's recall improve when prompting is provided?

    —is maximal cuing needed (providing choices, yes or no questions)?
    —is minimal cuing sufficient ("Wh" kinds of questions)?
    —is prodding sufficient ("Tell me more...")?

- Are medications affecting memory performance?

Strategies:

- For deficits in visual memory, teach the child to verbally encode information to be remembered.

- For deficits in verbal memory, teach visual imaging techniques for information to be remembered.
- Teach consistent use of logbooks or simple journals.
- Teach the child to map new information to easily remembered personal experiences, making strong associations to link the target information with previously stored and highly retrievable information.

9. *Judgment*:

- Does the child have basic safety awareness?
- Is his reaction time poor?
- Is there difficulty in making quick decisions?
- Does he attend to the environment with sufficient depth to notice potential danger?
- Does susceptibility to distraction make mobility in the community implausible?
- Does he consider the consequences of his behavior prior to acting or is he impulsive?
- Does he ask for advice he needs?

Strategies:

- Teach and habituate self-instructional questioning such as "Should I go ahead now" as a response to discriminative stimuli such as streets.
- Teach the child to carry and use simple written cues for problem situations.

10. *Behavior/Socialization*:

- Is the child appropriate or problematic in terms of being:

    — alert or lethargic?
    — goal-directed or a-motivated?
    — decisive or tentative?
    — inquiring or passive?
    — reflective or impulsive?
    — socially insightful or inhibited/disinhibited?
    — adjustive or inflexible to changes in routines?
    — emotionally stable or euphoric/depressed/labile?

- Is the child realistic in assessing his own task-performances?

- Can he accurately adjudge whether he has met a desired goal?
- Does he discern and react appropriately to nonverbal social cues such as facial expressions and voice tones?

Strategies:

- Teach the child to self-evaluate his behavior with specific questions relevant for specific goals.
- Teach self-reinforcement techniques for achievement of target behaviors.
- Teach deliberate scanning of facial expressions of others for cues to evaluate present behaviors.

These ten areas for conceptualizing cognition, their related clinical questions, and the compensatory strategies listed are by no means to be construed as complete. They are offered for guideline purposes of recognizing common behavioral patterns of head injured children, and for assistance in formulating goals for their treatment.

RELATED FUTURE TRENDS

The future will undoubtedly bring a greater understanding of cognition and its underlying principles than are reflected in the abovementioned considerations. The author and some of his co-workers in Cognitive Rehabilitation Therapy are hopeful that part of that understanding will include improved knowledge for the generalization of compensatory strategies. The current state of knowledge in that regard is lacking; more needs to be learned about how to effect carry-over of strategies mastered in treatment to the world at large. There is reason to be encouraged that future research will address such issues. Neisser (1982) is of the opinion that cognitive psychologists will increasingly concern themselves with issues and questions based less in the learning laboratories and more in functional settings. May he be clairvoyant.

There also promises to be continued research in the efficiency of direct treatment. Part of the goal of cognitive rehabilitation for head injured children has always been to channel spontaneous recovery, but the question of how much improvement was attributable to treatment and how much to spontaneous remission has remained largely unresolved. The issue may continue to be debated for some time. Meeting that question head-on could necessitate the provision of control groups who are not treated, raising immediate problems of ethics. But the matter of the effectiveness of treatment purporting both to stimulate appropriate and essential cortical activity and to teach the development of compensatory learning behaviors has caught the attention of increasing numbers of reputable minds. Ralph Reitan, mentioned at the beginning of this article, is one foremost among them. If he is representative of the level of research sophistication to be added to those already involved in treatment issues, then the impact should be felt for miles around and years to come.

There is the enormity of computer science to be considered as well. Cognitive rehabilitation is not, as some currently think, the total of the gadgetry being widely developed and used in various programs. The ramifications of this field into the maturing future of CRT will be sizeable, however, in ways perhaps currently only faintly imaginable. Cortical prostheses may be a contribution of computer science in the years ahead.

The future of this area of rehabilitation looks particularly exciting and hopeful, and the head injured children of the silent epidemic will be both a major focus and direct beneficiaries of that future. Having developed initially as a logical and needed extension of the neuropsychological-diagnostic effort, Cognitive Rehabilitation now appears to be firmly anchored under the umbrella of a growing Cognitive Science. So positioned, it is somewhat unique in its ability to function as both giver and receiver of knowledge in the interplay between theoretical and clinical settings. But of course its real value lies in its commitment to real-life children with real-life needs. Ralph Reitan's friend put it right: the essential question now is, "What are we going to do to help these people?" The answer looks to be something like, "We've got a good start and we can't help but learn more. Full speed ahead."

REFERENCES

Levin, H., Benton, A., & Grossman J., *Neurobehavioral consequences of closed head injury.* New York: Oxford University Press, 1982.

Malkmus, D., Booth, B. S., & Kadimer, C. *Rehabilitation of the head injured adult. Comprehensive cognitive management.* Professional Staff Association of Rancho Los Amigos Hospital, 1980.

Neisser, U. Memory observed. *Remembering in natural contexts.* San Francisco: W. H. Freeman & Company, 1982.

The Assessment of Cognitive Function for Use in Education

Harold W. Gordon, PhD

ABSTRACT. The dichotomy of cognitive function attributed to the right and left hemisphere of the brain is gaining popularity in its prospect for explaining learning disabilities, for application to classroom instruction and for new directions in education. While it is heartening to have one major field, education, benefit from the empirical endeavors of another, neuropsychology, the specter of over-simplification and worse, exploitation, has risen as a by-product of success. There are many positive signs that new insights to brain functions and organization will guide the teaching of our children and the remediation of educationally handicapped. But implications have been drawn before all the evidence is in. Research has provided lists of functions attributed to the left cerebral hemisphere such as "verbal," "sequential," "propositional," or "time dependent" and to the right hemisphere such as "spatial," "synthetic," "appositional," or "non-temporal." The transgression occurs in trying to explain and predict behavior by extrapolation from those terms without really understanding the evidence giving rise to them. Such "armchair" philosophy leads to errors and distortion.

The impact of neuropsychology on education is potentially rewarding, but scientific method of trial and evaluation must prevail to prevent discredit of both neuropsychology itself and those who seek to apply it to education. Our intention in this article is not to be exhaustive, but to outline the basis of our knowledge of hemispheric function, relate some of the first steps in its application to education, and highlight the implications and directions for further study.

Harold W. Gordon, Assistant Professor of Psychiatry, Western Psychiatric Institute and Clinic, 3811 O'Hara Street, Pittsburgh, PA 15213.

Experiments by the authors and the collaborators in this article were supported, in part, by a grant to Western Psychiatric Institute and Clinic, University of Pittsburgh, by the Richard King Mellon Foundation and a grant to Harold W. Gordon by the Heinz Foundation. Cooperation of The Korean Ministry of Education and the Pittsburgh Public Schools is gratefully acknowledged.

THE STUDY OF HEMISPHERIC SPECIALIZATION: SUITABLE SUBJECTS

Unilateral Lesion Patients

There are three subject groups in whom hemispheric specialization has been studied. The first, and in many ways most convenient, consists of patients with (verified) unilateral cortical lesions. In this group, the method is straightforward. A task is presented to patients with a lesion in the right hemisphere; the performance by this group is compared to performance on the same task by patients with a lesion in the left hemisphere (controlling for size, locus and cause of the lesion as well as age, sex, education, and handedness of the subject). The hypothesis is that hemispheric specialization for performance of these tasks will produce depressed performance in one of the lesioned groups but not the other. A decrement in performance by patients with a left (but not right) hemisphere lesion implies the left hemisphere had been needed, or rather, specialized, to perform that task. Conversely, had the right-lesioned group been deficient instead of the left, it would have been concluded the right hemisphere was necessary for the task. Discovering the cortical substrate related to performing a task is easy, the hard part is extracting the salient features of the task that *characterize* the cortical contribution. Was a task of facial recognition a skill of "spatial," "nonverbal," "analytic" or "pattern" processing? The danger of error lies in the synthesis of evidence, the attempt to combine all experimental results into a unifying scheme.

For patients with unilateral damage there is another problem. All conclusions are inferential; the evidence is circumstantial and negative. Research is unavoidably designed to discover what the lesioned group *cannot* perform and therefore force the conclusion, "had the cortex been undamaged, the patients could have done the task." More strongly, it is claimed that the area in which the cortex was damaged was the area in which the task is normally performed. This argument is flawed. A brain is not a stack of functional compartments individually operating to produce behavior. The brain is an integrated, multifunctional circuit working as a total system. Brain damage alters this system. A crude analogy would be a technician who causes a "buzz" in a television by removing a resistor from the circuit. The technician could not claim to have removed a "buzz suppressor." At best, the claim may be made that the audio portion was affected but not the video. Similar conclusions about brain function need corroboration by *positive* evidence offered by other techniques.

Non-Brain Damaged Subjects ("Normals")

The second group in whom investigations of hemispheric functions are carried out are normal (i.e., non-brain damaged) individuals. This group is, of course, the largest and most available to study. The experimental techniques are also many and varied. Asymmetries in hemispheric processing are inferred in the visual modality from differences in response time or accuracy to stimuli that are quick-flashed to the right or left visual fields. Similarly, hemispheric asymmetries are implied from differences in ear superiority in perception or recall of different auditory stimuli that are simultaneously presented to the left and right ears.

Other physiological and psychophysiological techniques, including electrodermal, electroencephalographic (evoked potential, alpha blocking, etc.), cerebral blood flow, lateral eye movement, and glucose metabolism, have all been used to confirm the notion of lateral asymmetries of function in normal subjects. To their credit, these studies provide positive evidence in support of the negative inferences inherent in the studies of patients with unilateral lesions. Thus while patients with right (posterior) damage are deficient in facial recognition, response times are faster (for recognition or recall) in the left visual field of normal subjects.

The major difficulty in interpreting results in normal subjects (other than the usual methodological problems) is that the right hemisphere is connected to the left hemisphere via massive nerve connections, the largest of which is called the corpus collosum. Interpretation must include the realization that hemispheric asymmetries are relative: functions are not *in* a specific hemisphere. At best, they are performed *relatively* better *by* a specific hemisphere. In fact there is no reason to assume functions are exclusively lateralized to one hemisphere or the other whether they are interconnected or not. Even if the two halves of the brain were divided, the left hemisphere may well be able to perform "right" hemisphere functions and the right hemisphere may perform "left" hemisphere functions. Indeed this is probably what happens most of the time.

Patients Requiring Surgical Brain Division

The separate investigation of specialized functions is theoretically most convenient to study in a third group of subjects— patients who, for alleviation of intractible epilepsy, have had all the cross-connections in the main part of the brain completely severed thereby dividing the brain into two, non-communicating halves or hemispheres. If one can confine stimuli to one hemisphere in these patients, information about processing in that hemisphere and that hemisphere alone can be investigated. The difficulty is guaranteeing that test instructions, response biases, and the like, do not favor one hemisphere or the other thereby clouding the interpretation of the performance of the task itself. For example, the right hemisphere cannot speak, so comparison of response based on verbal output would be meaningless.

One other cautionary measure in these patients is the neurological history. All patients who have undergone this surgery are suffering from epilepsy, so severe that medication was insufficient to control seizure activity. Therefore, all of the patients have brain damage with onsets at different ages, located in different locations and probably stemming from different causes. Meaningful information may be derived from these patients only insofar as existing lesions are inconsequential for interpretation of the results. Such may be the case if a *damaged* hemisphere is actually *better* at performing a particular task.

It is conceptually convenient to use the model of the divided brain to begin the study of the separate functions of the right and left hemispheres. These patients have provided the impetus for a host of studies (Sperry, 1982) in many directions. One of these directions has led to education, in general, and learning disabilities, in particular.

DISCOVERIES OF HEMISPHERIC SPECIALIZATION

The different kinds of hemispheric output was demonstrated dramatically soon after surgery by the brain-divided patients' superior ability of the right hand to write, while the left hand was superior in copying geometric figures (Bogen & Gazzaniga, 1965; Bogen, 1969). The left hand could not write even after "watching" the right hand perform, nor could the right hand draw after "watching" the right hand perform, nor could the right hand draw after "watching" the left hand perform. One is struck with the coexistence in the same cranium of two different, functionally independent cognitive centers. Whether the left hemisphere writes and the right draws in the normal individual is not known. But we do have preliminary evidence that the functional capacities of the two brain halves are different.

The words "analytic" and "synthetic" were applied to the left and right brains, respectively in another early experiment using a visual-tactual adaptation of the Spatial Relation subtest of the Differential Aptitude Test (Levy-Agresti & Sperry, 1968). In this experiment, the subject felt a wooden block out of sight and was required to select, from among 3 choices, the correct, unfolded, 2-dimensional representation. Not only was the left hand of the patient better at the task but it appeared to perform the task in a manner qualitatively different from that of the right. The left hand held the block almost without moving it, apparently trying "synthesize" the entire form. In contrast, the right hand serially felt each side of the block, one after the other, trying to "analyze" the parts. This apparent dichotomous strategy inspired the two terms.

There lies in this historical description a second lesson. We must understand how the descriptive terms are generated to properly understand the dichotomy of cognitive function. If the term "analytic" is to be applied to the left hemisphere, it must be remembered that it applies to the step-by-step, piecemeal analysis of the block in the above-described experiment. This conceptualization broadly fits the notion of sequential processing seen in other experiments (Carmon & Nachshon, 1971; Cohen, 1973). But validation of what might be meant by "analytic" has not been subsequently demonstrated.

Demonstration of right hemisphere specialization has been shown in further studies by the ability of the right hemisphere (of the brain-divided patients) to visualize (albeit through tactual presentation) a whole circle when given only an arc (Nebes, 1971), or visualize a completed geometric figure given an arrangement of its parts (Nebes, 1972). One term applied to this ability is "closure." Tactually presented geometric figures were also better recognized by the left hand (D. Zaidel & Sperry, 1973; Franco & Sperry, 1977). Thus far we can attach words such as "synthetic," "wholistic" (from the ability in closure) and "pattern perceiver" to the list of right hemisphere characteristics. Other characteristics have been described in studies with unilateral lesions and in normals including superior right hemisphere performance for recognition of nonsense shapes, directionality (left/right, inverted/non-inverted), and locating points in space. (For a review, see De Renzi, 1982).

Language, speech in particular, is the dominant cognitive activity of the left hemisphere even though comprehension abilities are also found for the right hemisphere (E. Zaidel, 1978). But in addition, temporality or sequencing has been attributed to the left hemisphere. Left dominance is implied from deficits in aphasics for the judgment of simultaneity (Efron, 1963) and for the perception of temporal ordering in non-aphasic patients with left hemisphere lesions (Carmon & Nachshon, 1971). Left hemisphere processing is further confirmed in intact subjects where auditory stimuli are presented temporally (Halperin, Nachshon, & Carmon, 1973) or rhythmically (Gordon, 1978). Visual sequencing also appears to be left hemisphere dominant (Horan, Ashton, & Minto, 1980) although mixed results may indicate the presence of a spatial element as well (De Renzi, Faglioni, & Villo, 1977; Kim, Royer, Boustello & Boller, 1980).

ASSESSMENT OF COGNITIVE FUNCTION AND ITS USE

These research studies are what give a fairly clear idea of what kinds of tasks are performed better by the right hemisphere and which are performed better by the left. Based on these characteristics it is common to observe that some people appear to perform tasks associated with left hemisphere processes better than they perform tasks associated with the right hemisphere. Others perform tasks associated with right hemisphere processes better than they perform tasks associated with right hemisphere processes better than they perform tasks associated with the left. While these observations may be true, it does not necessarily follow that such people have a dominant, or more active, left hemisphere or a dominate or more active right hemisphere. In fact, attempts to demonstrate this point have failed (Arndt & Berger, 1978). The leap from research delineating *where* in the normal brain certain functions are located does not predict *how* the normal brain will contribute to day-to-day performance of that behavior. A "left hemisphere person," defined as one who performs better on functions attributed to the left hemisphere, may be performing these primarily "left brain" functions from both sides of the cerebrum. Research on this point is incomplete.

There is no "normal" degree of hemisphericity—the amount of cognitive skill produced by each hemisphere, just as for "intelligence" the norm has to be determined empirically. Accordingly, a battery of tests (The Cognitive Laterality Battery) was designed to assess the relative performance on abilities attributed to the right and left cerebral hemispheres. (A full description and manual are in preparation; see also Gordon, 1983.) A cognitive profile is defined as the relation between performance on right hemisphere tests to performance on left hemisphere tests. Since the tests have been standardized, a "normal" performance is defined as equal performance (contribution) from each hemisphere: no asymmetry. The cognitive profile would be determined from the difference between performance on tests attributed to the right hemisphere and tests attributed to the left hemisphere.

The K-ABC: Kaufman Assessment Battery for Children (A. Kaufman & N. Kaufman, 1983) is an already-published "intelligence" test based on the same neuropsychological principles as the CLB. The subtests may be categorized into a "sequential" and "simultaneous" grouping for comparison. The K-ABC is primarily for use with younger children. The norms range from age 2½ to 12. However, it must be administered individually with a trained tester, while the CLB is designed as a group-administered test but has been standardized only from the 4th grade through adult. While such test administrations are state-of-the-art, the advent of microcomputers will soon revolutionize testing and testing methods. The number of individuals that can be tested at one time will be limited only by the number of computer terminals. Testers will not need special training; scoring will be done automatically. More importantly, tests may be devised such that the testee may interact with the test. In this way an examiner may gain insight to the *way* in which problems are being solved, not just the final scores. This is exactly what the CLB and K-ABC are trying to accomplish in their crude form. It is the *type* of thinking that is the aim of the cognitive tests in the first place.

The new contribution of these tests and ones like them is that the assessment is closer to the brain processes themselves. Cognitive testing gives a qualitative picture—a cognitive profile—of a person's strengths or weaknesses. Instead of a "vertical" dimension of who is better and who is worse on a test, a "horizontal" dimension of relative performance between two kinds of thinking is produced.

Learning Disabled

A prime candidate for application of cognitive tests is the child with a learning disability. Evidence has been accruing for some time that an asymmetry of cognitive performance is common in such individuals. One of the consistent findings is a deficit for the perception or processing of sequences (Bakker, 1967). Sequencing, as we have pointed out, is attributed to functioning of the left hemisphere. Of course, deficits in verbal expression and phonological decoding (Vellutino, 1978) are always associated with learning difficulties; these functions are also attributed to the left hemisphere. Conversely, normal, if not above normal, performances on visual-spatial tasks are reported for these individuals. A quick check of Digit Span (especially digits forward) in comparison to Block Design will reveal consistent asymmetries where Block Design is performed better than Digit Span by almost 3 scaled points (1.0 standard deviation) (Naidoo, 1972). The same asymmetry has been reported in another grouping of the subtests. A Spatial category made up of Object Assembly, Block Design, and Picture Completion was always performed better than a Sequential category made up of Digit Span, Picture Arrangement and Coding (Rugel, 1974). The difference was, again nearly 1.0 standard deviation.

To assess the cognitive profile of such individuals, the Cognitive Laterality Battery was administered to a year's worth of referrals to a reading disability clinic after being screened for definite neurological signs of brain damage and mental retardation. Out of 108 subjects nearly all, 105, had performed better on tests of right hemisphere functions than on tests of left. The average differences was more than 1.0 standard deviation which is not only substantial, but also close to the magnitude already observed for the Block Design/Digit Span differences.

It is probably not a surprise that learning disabled individuals tend to be relatively better on visual-spatial tasks (or at least, worse on sequential/verbal tasks), although the percentage of subjects with this asymmetry may have been surprising. What was unexpected, however, was that the performance on tests attributed to the right hemisphere was about 0.5 standard deviation *above aver-*

age as compared to age-matched controls. Our data seem to be saying that the same individuals who have a deficiency in one or more of their cognitive functions have a superiority in another.

This evidence seems to suggest that a cognitive profile favoring right hemisphere tests is characteristic of virtually all or a very high percentage of learning-disabled individuals. This conclusion is premature. The subject selection was limited: a more exhaustive selection would undoubtedly have produced more subjects with cognitive profiles favoring left hemisphere tests. A second, limitation to placing individuals along a right/left hemisphere continuum is that it masks the possible existence of subtypes. Even though 97% of the subjects performed better on tests of right hemisphere function, they still may be subgrouped further on other cognitive measures. For some purposes, then, it is better to consider a broader range of learning-disabled individuals, in which there will be one or two "left hemisphere" subtypes and several "right hemisphere" subtypes.

TESTING CHILDREN UNIDENTIFIED FOR LEARNING DIFFICULTIES

In spite of the possibility that some dyslexics may have a task preference favoring the left hemisphere, it does seem safe to conclude that a majority of learning-disabled subjects perform better on tests of right hemisphere function. It appears, therefore, that for most learning-disabled individuals, the cognitive profile favoring the right hemisphere is a *necessary* condition for the learning deficit. Of course, not all individuals who perform relatively better on tests of right hemisphere function are learning-disabled, so the profile is not *sufficient*. Nevertheless, it is reasonable to hypothesize that individuals with a right hemisphere preference will be *at risk* for learning difficulties, especially on achievement tests.

This idea has been substantiated on two elementary and middle school populations, one in Korea (750 subjects) and one in a major urban school district (1100 subjects). The CLB was administered to classroom-size groups whose cognitive profile was calculated on age- and sex-appropriate norms (Koh, 1982; Gordon, in preparation). The subjects were divided into 2 groups according to whether they performed better on "right" or "left" tests. The performances of the 2 groups were compared on each of a number of standard achievement tests. Those that performed better on right tests (a "right" hemisphericity) were consistently and significantly worse than those with a "left" hemisphericity on most measures of language and reading, even when levels of overall performance were co-varied with the profile scores. In other words, any differences among the subjects in intellectual capacity did not explain the group differences. Furthermore, when the right/left groups were subdivided into below-average and above-average subgroups, it was the above-average "right" and "left" hemisphericity groups that differed more significantly between themselves. The important lesson to be learned from these data is that intellectual capabilities alone are not good predictors of achievement scores. An evaluator—teacher, counselor, principal—must take into consideration a child's cognitive profile as well.

EXTENDING THE CONCEPT OF COGNITIVE ASSESSMENT TO SCHOOL CURRICULA

Neuropsychologists who believe in the qualitative differences of cognitive function, may informally classify people along the right/left continuum as "right hemisphere" thinkers and "left hemisphere" thinkers. There is some validation that this difference is meaningful for some adult occupations. For example, fighter pilots have better performance on right tests than helicopter pilots (Gordon, Silverberg-Shalev & Czernilas, 1982). But we do not know how a child's thinking style helps or hinders learning in matched or unmatched curricula. Educated guesses could well be made, but the evidence is lacking.

It has been encouraging that some preliminary data point in the correct direction. Normal high school students who performed better on the summed Verbal, Numerical, and the Clerical subtests of the Differential Aptitude Tests than on the Mechanical Reasoning subtest performed relatively better on left hemisphere tests. Those whose performance on these subtests was reversed had the right hemisphere cognitive profile. In another small study (Gordon, 1979; Gordon, 1983) gifted elementary children who participated (by choice) in an extracurricular "model building" class performed better on right hemisphere (than on left hemisphere) tests while those who participated in a creative writing class performed better on the left hemisphere tests.

Nevertheless, before we put our "right hemisphere" children into art, music, geometry and carpentry classes and our "left hemisphere" children into history, rhetoric, and trigonometry classes, we need to be cautious and patient until the validation data have been collected in appropriately-controlled studies. There is no evidence that teaching with methods or materials conducive to right hemisphere thinking has ever enhanced or developed the right hemisphere's inherent ability, whether it happened to be the individual's weaker hemisphere or stronger hemisphere. The same is true for left hemisphere methods. There is, as yet, no evidence on which to decide whether a learning disabled child with a large asymmetry favoring the right hemisphere should have remedial instruction that exploits the good right hemisphere, exercises the weak left hemisphere, or combines the two. Only when the three methods are compared, side by side, in three equivalent teaching situations can a decision be made. Currently, the state of the art is to be able to assess hemisphericity with good reliability and validity and to use this assessment for understanding the relative capabilities—the cognitive profiles—of children. We have learned that intellectual capacity of an individual is only part of the picture. It is probably a good idea to extend the teaching curriculum to include development and training of all basic brain functions including the special functions of the right and left hemispheres; it has to be better than teaching half the brain. Continued research in neuropsychology promises to be fruitful for payoff in education. But patience and cooperation among different academic disciplines will prevent steps backward in work that has only just begun.

REFERENCES

Arndt, A., & Berger, D. E. Cognitive mode and asymmetry in cerebral functioning. *Cortex*, 1978, *14*, 78-86.

Bakker, D. J. Temporal order, meaningfulness, and reading ability. *Perceptual & Motor Skills*, 1967, *24*, 1027-1030.

Bogen, J. E. The other side of the brain, I. Dysgraphia and dyscopia following cerebral commissurotomy. *Bulletin of the Los Angeles Neurological Societies*, 1969, *34*, 73-105.

Bogen, J. E., & Gazzaniga, M. S. Cerebral commissurotomy in man. Minor hemisphere dominance for certain visuospatial functions. *Journal of Neurosurgery*, 1965, *23* (4), 394-399.

Carmon, A., & Nachshon, I. Effect of unilateral brain damage on perception of temporal order. *Cortex*, 1971, *7*, 410-418.

Cohen, G. Hemispheric differences in serial versus parallel processing. *Journal of Experimental Psychology*, 1973, *97*(3), 349-356.

DeRenzi, E. *Disorders of Space Exploration and Cognition.* New York: John Wiley & Sons, 1982.

DeRenzi, E., Faglioni, P., & Villa, P. Sequential memory for figures in brain-damaged patients. *Neuropsychologia,* 1977, *15,* 43-49.

Franco, L., & Sperry, R. W. Hemisphere lateralization for cognitive processing of geometry. *Neuropsychologia,* 1977, *15,* 107-114.

Gordon, H. W. Left hemisphere dominance for rhythm elements in dichotically-presented melodies. *Cortex,* 1978, *14,* 58-70.

Gordon, H. W. Right and left hemisphere thinking in gifted children. Presented at the 3rd International Conference on Gifted and Talented Children. Jerusalem, Israel, 1979.

Gordon, H. W. The right style of the learning disabled. In M. Kinsbourne (Ed.), *Topics in Learning and Learning Disabilities,* 1983, *3*(1), 29-39.

Gordon, H. W., Silverberg-Shalev, R., & Czernilas, J. Hemispheric asymmetry in fighter and helicopter pilots. *Acta Psychologica,* 1982, 52, 33-40.

Halperin, Y., Nachshon, I., & Carmon, A. Shift of ear superiority in dichotic listening to temporally patterned nonverbal stimuli. *J. Acoust. Soc. Am.,* 1973, *53*(1), 46-50.

Horan, M., Ashton, R., & Minto, J. Using ECT to study hemispheric specialization for sequential processes. *British Journal of Psychiatry,* 1980, *137,* 119-125.

Kaufman, A., & Kaufman, N. K-ABC: The Kaufman Assessment Battery for Children. Circle Pines, Mm: American Guidance Service, 1983.

Kim, Y., Royer, F., Boustelle, C., & Boller, F. Temporal sequencing of verbal and nonverbal materials: The effect of laterality of lesion. *Cortex,* 1980, *16,* 135-143.

Levy-Agresti, J., & Sperry, R. W. Differential perceptual capacities in major and minor hemispheres. *Proceedings of the National Academy of Science,* 1968, *61,* 1151.

Naidoo, S. *Specific Dyslexia.* New York: John Wiley & Sons, 1972.

Nebes, R. D. Superiority of the minor hemisphere in commissurotomized man for the perception of part-whole relations. *Cortex,* 1971, *7,* 333-349.

Nebes, R. D. Dominance of the minor hemisphere in commissurotomized man on a test of figural unification. *Brain,* 1972, *95*(III), 633-638.

Rugel, R. P. WISC Subtest scores of disabled readers: A review with respect to Bannatyne's recategorization. *Journal of Learning Disabilities,* 1974, *7*(1), 48-65.

Sperry, R. W. Some effects of disconnecting the cerebral hemispheres. (Nobel presentation) *Science,* 1982, *217,* 1223-1226.

Vellutino, F. R. Toward an understanding of dyslexia: Psychological factors in specific reading disability. In A. L. Benton, & D. Pearl (Eds.), *Dyslexia:* An Appraisal of Current Knowledge. New York: Oxford University Press, 1978.

Zaidel, D., & Sperry, R. W. Performance on the Raven's colored progressive matrices test by subjects with cerebral commissurotomy. *Cortex,* 1973, *9,* 34-39.

Zaidel, E., Lexical organization in the right hemisphere. In P. Buser, & A. Rougel-Buser (Eds.), *Cerebral Correlates of Conscious Experience,* INSERM Symposium No. 6. Amsterdam: Elsevier/North Holland Biomedical Press, 1978.

The Impact of Brain Research on the Education Profession: Agents of Change

David B. Straham, EdD
Conrad F. Toepfer, Jr., EdD

ABSTRACT. The neuroscience knowledge explosion is organizing a critical data base on how the brain works and functions. Brain research findings can help identify how and when children can develop more sophisticated intellectual skills. This seems important for re-thinking effective school practice. Since educators lack neurological training and neurologists lack pedagogic background, a base to organize such data must be developed. Educational psychology has long been a foundational area for pedagogical development. The syncretizing of neurological data on brain function with psychological theories of learning could organize a *neuropsychology of learning*. From this base, curriculum developers could plan educational programs which respond to developmental capacities to think and process information.

Characteristics of seven areas of development are offered as a base for developing such a neuropsychological foundation area. Theory and present practice in several areas are suggested for rethinking current educational practice. The beginning use of computers to match teaching and learning at different developmental stages in children is also discussed. As educators develop agents of change to improve school curricula, the degree to which those efforts respond to developmental thinking capacities will be critical.

David B. Straham is Assistant Professor in the Department of Elementary and Secondary Education and Reading at State University College, Geneseo, NY 14454. Conrad F. Toepfer, Jr. is Associate Professor in the Department of Learning and Instruction, State University of New York at Buffalo, Buffalo, NY 14260.

CHANGES AND CHALLENGES

Changes

Public confidence in educational innovation has lessened since the decade of the 1960s. The phasing in and out of rafts of innovations during those years was rapid. Many promising innovations were aborted before impact could be determined. Others were cut short either because of lack of continued funding or newer "fads." This promoted increasing cynicism over "change for the sake of change" and markedly lowered the credibility of new educational departures among both public and professional constituencies. Contemporary skepticism of educational change has crystallized a "back-to-basics" focus through the report of the National Commission on Excellence in Education (Gardner, 1983.) The "Nation at Risk" report has championed the need to improve achievement in basic skill areas such as language, mathematics, and science by extending traditional subject matter approaches. This emphasis has developed at a time when increased public and professional awareness of popularized reporting of the current explosion in the neurosciences is also surfacing.

Challenge

The lack of sophisticated neurological training among both lay and educator groups make it imperative that no quantum change from present school practice be made on mere casual assumptions of new understandings. The challenge includes: the consideration of known realities of what learning is and how it takes place against the emerging data on how the brain functions; the study of how children develop and mature thinking capacities during their journey through childhood and the years of schooling; the principles of effective curriculum planning must be strictly followed if any real improvement of educational experience in terms of brain research data is to be achieved.

It is important to include the education of parents and the lay public to the reality of children's educational needs as such a lack of public understanding has undoubtedly contributed to the abortion of many promising educational advances. Any chance for reasonable success in school programs responding to neurological realities must include a strategy for lay orientation.

TOWARD A NEUROPSYCHOLOGY OF EDUCATION

Previous mention was made of the lack of neuroscience background among professional educators. Teachers, administrators, counselors, school psychologists and curriculum planners all are largely ignorant of such information in their formal, professional education. As was also stated, educational psychology is the discipline from which educators learn about learning. Theories of learning, experimental data on learning and the relationship of child development to learning approaches are studied in educational psychology. This, then, is the foundational area from which educators base the theory and practice of teaching and learning for curriculum and program development. The area of educational psychology appears to be the best source for establishing an interface with the neuroscience data base which educators currently lack. However, consider the horns of this dilemma as it presently exists.

The lack of neuroscience background among educators is paralleled in that neuroscientists interested in applying their findings to educational and learning settings have a virtual universal ignorance in areas such as curriculum planning and development. While organizing teams of neuroscientists, educational psychologists and curriculum planners could establish a base for interfacing these data bases, no continuing solution would be achieved. As Toepfer suggests (1982), such efforts would provide a basis for developing a neuropsychology of education which could become the primary foundational area for educational preparation and development. This would establish an arena for the interaction of neuroscience findings with theories of learning and child development. Existing areas of learning theory could gain both specification and validation which could improve teaching-learning settings beyond levels currently not possible. This syncretism of educational psychology and neuroscience into a neuropsychology of learning would provide a major foundational area of study for all educators. It would facilitate the cooperative efforts of curriculum planners with neuropsychologically competent learning theorists. This could result in learning activities which respond to the developmental capacities of children to think and learn across the years of schooling.

Areas of Achievement to Date

Neuroscience research and renewed interest in cognitive development have produced a proliferation of ideas for assessing and teaching thinking in learners. National and regional conferences have offered a wide array of programs disseminating information on growth patterns, thought processes, testing procedures, teaching strategies, and student activities. In a variety of publications, researchers have offered new instruments for measuring cognitive growth, described various modes of thinking, suggested numerous formal and informal observation procedures, and presented frameworks for analyzing curricular requirements with respect to levels of thinking. This proliferation of ideas from research and practice now provides a data base from which educators can begin to plan and develop more systematic and integrated curricula and learning activities. As more teachers become aware of the need to teach thinking skills, curriculum planners will need to explore ways to integrate thinking enrichment more effectively with content instruction. This will be essential to the planning of programs which encourage development of thinking more holistically. Hopefully, a neuropsychology of learning will combine information on learning theory with data on brain function so that programs will respond to how children think and learn as they grow and mature. The total spectrum of our educational establishment needs to study these possibilities.

SEVEN ESSENTIAL CHARACTERISTICS

While "integration" (Hopkins, 1937; Krug, 1950) has long been a goal of curriculum planners and a hallmark of educational philosophies, recent insights from research on brain function and thought processes provide additional support for needs to develop integrated instructional approaches. This is all the more critical as psychological data confirm the developmental nature of learning. If children are to develop new modes of thinking and processing information as they grow and mature, school programs and learning activities must become developmentally responsive to their increasing readiness. Such research suggests the following seven essential characteristics of an integrated approach to improve teaching for thinking. These characteristics are an attempt to present the highlights of research on brain functions that relates to classroom thinking and curricular planning. As such, they may provide a preliminary framework for designing more detailed guidelines for constructing curricula, conducting evaluation, and providing inservice programs. When considered together, these characteristics provide an overview of an integrated approach to thinking enrichment and a strong rationale for systematic, guided instruction throughout our educational system.

Acknowledgment of the Complexities of Thinking

As neuroscientists discover new information about the brain, appreciation of the complexities of thinking grows. Comparing the brain to "a chemical computer with circuits whirring with both electricity and chemicals," Begley, Carey, and Sawhill (1983) assert that "the brain has always been and will always be more complicated than man's latest contraption. . . . It sends neuroscientists where no researcher has ever explored before" (p. 42). One dimension of this complexity is what Hart (1982) calls "the brain's overwhelming numbers." Noting that there may be as many as 30 billion neurons in the brain, some with as many as 10,000 connections with other neurons, Hart suggests that "as we perceive the possible combinations beyond the trillions, we can begin to grasp why the brain can be so subtle—and why each brain is so different from any other" (p. 198). Another dimension of the complexity of thinking is the discoveries about individual variations in brain "blueprints." Ojemann (1983) discovered, for example, that some subjects' sites for naming objects lie in the parietal lobes while other subjects' sites are more numerous in the temporal lobes. While speculations emerge about brain organization and intelligence, it seems clear that there are many ways for the brain to organize information. Given the astronomical "numbers" involved in thinking and the apparent individual variation in organizing and storing information, teachers should beware of attempts to oversimplify thought processes or to reduce thinking to simple taxonomies or skills lists.

Emphasis on Analogical as Well as Logical Thinking

While much of the attention in encouraging thinking has been focused upon concrete and formal operations and the development of "higher order" reasoning, a number of learning theorists caution against undue emphasis on logic. Eisner (1981) suggests that over-emphasis on the role of logic in cognition has limited educators' views of thinking processes. He suggests that crucial sensory, perceptual, and imaginative operations are necessary to form concepts as well as logical operations. Sherman (1979) notes that "the true scientist makes his intuitive leaps and imaginative thrusts into regions beyond the explicit and verbalizable" (p. 9). Levin (1976) reports a series of studies describing the critical role of "visual imagery" in middle grades students' thinking, noting the analogical nature of such imagery even while performing prose comprehension tasks. Strahan (1982) also discovered a relatively high frequency of "visualization" responses to seemingly logical problem-solving tasks. While Levy (1982) and others have noted that the "right brain/left brain" differential is not nearly as straightforward as once believed, different dimensions of thinking certainly exist and interact. Thinking enrichment efforts must thus encourage experiences with a wide variety of thinking, including image-mediated activities, artistic endeavors, and visual imagery strategies.

Emphasis on Nonverbal as Well as Verbal Learning

Recent investigations of "right brain/left brain" thinking have also emphasized the importance of nonverbal learning as well as analogical learning. Sinatra (1983) reports a series of such investigations and states a strong case for the importance of nonverbal learning in both language development and conceptual learning. One study (Glassner, 1980) is especially illustrative. Using an EEG procedure which allowed researchers to study the actual engagement of the two hemispheres during cognitive tasks, researchers analyzed students' thinking during two different modes of writing—conveying a message and expressing feelings. Results demonstrate that while the writing product is linear, writing processes incorporate nonverbal and nonlinear modes of thinking. Haglund (1981) also reviews a range of research in verbal and nonverbal learning and suggests that teachers prepare students in conceptual awareness of facts before introducing abstract symbols, guide students in image-mediated thinking, allow students choices in regard to methods of receiving and reporting information, and encourage awareness of learning styles. While activities that enrich nonverbal learning seem especially necessary, so too are speaking and listening. Hart (1975) notes that while a significant portion of the neocortex is structured toward oral language and that "thinking aloud" is necessary to the expansion of neural capacity, many school activities stress reading and writing. Given this seemingly paradoxical demand for both verbal and nonverbal experiences, teachers are once again encouraged to plan varied and experiential learning activities. As summarized by Levy (1982),

> As the child learns to read, communicate orally, learn history, or engage in any other so-called 'verbal activity,' both sides of his or her brain are learning, being educated, participating in the growth of understanding. The child's appreciation of literature depends on his or her ability to synthesize letters into words, words into sentences, sentences into meaning and thought. It depends on the ability to apprehend and respond to the rhythm of language; to imagine and feel the scenes and moods; to empathize with the characters and understand their emotions, values and personalities; and to integrate all this into a rich and full meaning with structure, configuration, and detail. (p. 176)

Emphasis on Horizontal Enrichment as Well as Vertical Enrichment

Among the many insights to emerge from Piaget's research is the fundamental notion that children develop new modes of thinking through wide ranging experiences with operations at their existing level. This emphasis on "horizontal" enrichment characterizes many of the attempts to "match" curricular activities with levels of thinking. Research in brain growth periodization suggests that new synaptic connections form during growth spurt periods, creating a neurological base for cognitive maturation. The danger of overloading students with excessive "vertical" enrichment has been documented dramatically in Toepfer's research on the "turn off phenomenon" (1981). Evidence from numerous brain studies suggests clearly portions of the neocortex "shut down" when faced with undue stress, impeding, shrinking and limiting performance

(Hart, 1975). Providing horizontal enrichment and limiting undue stress does not require rigid avoidance of unfamiliar or more abstract thinking activities, however. On the contrary, Piaget strongly stressed the need for exposure to varied cognitive tasks, for verbal interactions, and for some degree of challenge. Levy (1982) strongly underscores the need for challenge, suggesting that "challenges are what appear to engage the whole brain, to generate excitement and interest and attention, to provide the substrate for optimal learning" (p. 182). Evidence suggests that when tasks are simple, bilateral activation is at a low level. The brain seems to rely on one hemisphere, receiving little facilitation from the other side. If this is the case, active learning can only result when the whole brain is aroused and engaged, suggesting that teachers try to provide meaningful challenge without overload.

Ongoing Assessment of Student Thinking Using a Range of Formal and Informal Procedures

Almost all attempts to relate research on brain growth to classroom practices involve some systematic assessment of students' levels and styles of thinking. What seems to be essential is ongoing observation at the classroom level. In reporting their work on "Cognitive Levels Matching," Brooks, Fusco, and Grennon (1983) note that "assessing the cognitive levels of students involves both an analytic understanding of students' questions and responses in daily interactions in the classroom, as well as use of more formal techniques" (p. 6). Formal techniques used in their program are clinical methods with the traditional Piagetian tasks and the newly developed Arlin Test of Formal Reasoning (1982). These formal measures are used to supplement and support teacher observations. Given the growing array of formal and informal measures for assessing thinking, teachers should carefully select those measures that fit their situation and studiously observe student responses to thinking enrichment activities.

Ongoing Analysis of the Cognitive Demands of Required Tasks

In order to provide varied thinking enrichment activities and to integrate thinking enrichment with content instruction, teachers must become proficient in analyzing the cognitive demands of classroom tasks. As described in detail by Elkind (1980):

Accordingly, task analysis of necessity looks at the form (the complexity of instructions, illustrations, format) as well as the content (the concepts, materials, examples) of curriculum materials. It tries to determine what level of reasoning is demanded by a given curriculum material (its logical substructure) and whether that level of reasoning is appropriate to the age group being served. (p. 21)

Such analysis, coupled with ongoing observation of students as they interact with selected materials and activities, is the essential core of integrated enrichment. Unless the teacher clearly understands what the activity demands of the student, it will be impossible to plan appropriate guided instruction.

Guided Instruction in Developing More Abstract Concepts in Content Subjects

The process of guided instruction brings together everything that the teacher knows about students' thinking and the nature of the content subject itself. Ongoing assessment using formal and informal measures provides information about the levels and processes of students' thinking. Ongoing content analysis provides information about the levels of abstraction and cognitive demands of the content materials. All of this information now provides a basis for planning lesson strategies that can both teach content and thinking skills. While a wide range of strategies have been developed over the years, research on thinking processes underscores the necessity for systematic instruction and suggests two essential elements in such instruction:

a. varied experiences combining logical/analogical and verbal/nonverbal enrichment activities.
b. systematic progression from present experiences toward more advanced interpretations.

As suggested above, learners need horizontal thinking enrichment activities in order to generate more complex ideas. This is also necessary as the learner uses his or her readiness to move on to new and more difficult thinking activities. Guided instruction is primarily the process of selecting critical ideas from content subjects and helping students build to those ideas through varied thinking and learning experiences.

TASKS AND MEANS FOR CHANGE

Education faces its greatest need in taking what a neuropsychology of learning can provide to the critical areas of pre-service education of teachers and other professionals as well as in-service education of present educators. The seven essential characteristics previously discussed as well as the other pieces in this journal suggest both theoretical and operational indications of what substance for that change may be. Models for both pre- and in-service programs can presently be developed. The major problem shall, of course, be the perennial political one. Vested interests of traditionalists, subject matter specialists, "back-to-basics" advocates and others, all need to be educated to what brain research identifies. As fears are allayed and it is made clear that subject matter and basics can be more effectively learned through teaching to readiness patterns which neuropsychology establishes as true, definitive progress can be made. Attempts to develop new programs prior to that understanding shall have limited chances for success.

Re-thinking of existing teaching methodology courses along developmental facts will be a major project. Not only is the use of testing to identify cognitive readiness, hemispheric, higher brain function and other variables crucial, the need is also to prepare educators who can assess their own teaching for its appropriateness in those dimensions. Development of appropriate instructional materials, units of study and preparation of teachers to interact with students at appropriate levels must be central elements in teacher education and re-education programs. Careful efforts in these areas can develop means to achieve substantial improvement in making private and public elementary, middle level and high school programs responsive to the developmental capacities of learners.

It seems evident that post-secondary schools, especially colleges and universities will have a major responsibility in developing such programs. Colleges of education, medical schools, science and psychology departments will combine their research, teaching and dissemination systems for the education of school personnel and development of materials. However, what are the needs to improve the effectiveness and responsiveness in the collegiate institution itself? The issue of professors as teachers rather than lecturers has long been a concern to all but the professors. The degree to which post-secondary institutions will face up to this reality is not promising as measured by past history. However, any evaluation of the effectiveness or responsiveness of college instruction indicates major needs for change. If considered, the neurosciences offer as great a potential for improving instruction at community college, undergraduate and graduate institutions as at lower levels.

Your authors here have sought to examine ways of dealing with future application of the present stage of development in neurologically-psychologically based educational efforts. As stated, the full potential of such efforts shall rely upon the articulated development of a neuropsychological foundations area for educational and curriculum planning. However, three aspects of the "state-of-the-art" stand as data sources which can be studied for use by schools and educators. They offer means to specify the tasks faced in dealing with the issues presented in this article.

1. Cognitive Levels Matching

The work of Epstein (1974, 1978, 1979, 1981) in the area of brain growth periodization was foundational to the development of cognitive levels matching programs. Sylwester's piece in this journal carefully synthesizes that work for educators. Brooks, Fusco and Grennon (1983) and Fusco in this journal cite the encouraging state of attempts to match learning and teaching on changing cognitive levels.

Established Piagetian testing instruments for children between ages 2 and 10 years have long supported efforts to identify cognitive levels during that childhood age frame. Efforts to extend cognitive levels matching for students from the age 11-18 years frame relied on more recent attempts in assessment. Beginning testing efforts to assess cognitive levels during that age interval were initiated by Ankney and Joyce (1976), Burney (1976), and Lawson (1978). Arlin (1982) (also see this journal) has refined testing which identifies cognitive levels for the age 11-18 age group. As the sources cited here identify, efforts at effective cognitive levels matching in assessment and teaching are progressing to levels from which guidelines for adaptation and development in other school settings can be anticipated.

2. Left/Right/Whole Brain Thinking

While Levy (1982) warns against trying to identify left and right brain curricula, the data on learning styles and hemispheric dominance should cause educators to examine current school practice. Bogen (1975), Gazzaniga (1974), Kinsbourne and Hiscock (1978), and Riegel (1979), provide a data base against which we can assess present school practice and curriculum organization. Toepfer (1982) considers areas of traditional school practice to be biased against right brain dominant learners. Traditional schooling tasks favor linear, sequential, analytical and logical operations which are strengths of left hemisphere dominant learners. Right brain dominant learners who excel at spatial, holistic, visual spatial tactile and intuitive have much greater difficulty in meeting curriculum and learning challenges which are contrary to their right hemisphere dominance.

Educators need to explore ways in which traditional learning areas can be offered in styles and modes of processing more common to right brain dominant learners. McCarthy (1982) has developed approaches to identify brain dominance using left/right modes to teach to individual learner needs. Reynolds (1982) cautions about the problems in assessing hemispheric dominance. However, the testing pioneered by Torrance (1977) can be improved only as these instruments continue to be used and refined.

3. Computers

As schools meet the critical need to provide teachers with computer literacy at basic assembly language levels, the micro-computer can provide tactical means to the ends considered under the two previous points. The user-friendly LOGO computer language with its "turtle-talk" capacity has proven workable even with early childhood learners. Lough (1983a, 1983b) discusses the application of LOGO programs to right and left brain modes. Carter (1983) identifies the capacity of LOGO to work at different cognitive levels. It would be possible, for instance, to teach the same content statement to students at differing cognitive levels using LOGO language with a micro-computer. This opens the way to learners seeking their appropriate level of learning and thinking by choosing from the alternatives which the computer can present. The potential for motivating learners to seek their optimal level at a given age as well as to work across the spectrum of thinking levels which they have achieved is exciting. The mobility of computer graphics for visual-spacial preferences of more right brain dominant learners also offers a rich potential. The most hopeful consideration is that it will take teachers who have learned how to develop computer programs which can achieve this. Thus the goal of teachers able to plan more responsive learning activities for students may be be assisted through teacher interaction with the computer to plan diversified individual and small group learning activities. As we learn more of what the neurosciences identify as systems and function of the brain, computer programming can synthesize the levels and styles of individual learners. While it augurs hard work it also augurs an exciting means to achieve responsive learning opportunities.

CONCLUSION

Both the possibilities and probabilities suggested here and others not considered are streaking toward us at accelerating speeds. The knowledge explosion in our civilization currently means a total turnover and doubling of information every two-and-a-half years. We no longer live in an environment in which learning and memorization of facts provide a virtual constant data base for our lives. While facts, information and skills still are at the center of the teaching-learning act, our knowledge data bases will change and increase more frequently. Perhaps the very survival of our species depends on how well we educate our youth as effective thinkers. We can think of no other agenda more important for educators than the effectiveness with which we come to understand what the neurosciences are telling us about how the brain functions. As we can learn and understand those data, keep abreast of the growth and change in that data base and interface it with our knowledge of learning and child development, we may increase the odds on winning the age old race between education and disaster!

REFERENCES

Ankney, P., & Joyce, L. Concrete-operational reasoning test. In R. B. Sund (Ed.), *Piaget for educators*. Columbus, Ohio: Charles E. Merrill Publishing Company, 1976, 154-164.

Arlin, P. K. *The Arlin test of formal reasoning*. Unpublished test under revision. Vancouver: University of British Columbia, 1982.

Begley, S., Carey, J., & Sawhill, R. How the brain works. *Newsweek,* February 7, 1983, 42.

Bogen, J. Some educational aspects of hemispheric specialization, *UCLA Educator,* Spring, 1975, *17,* 24-32.

Brooks, M., Fusco, E., & Grennon, J. Cognitive levels matching. *Educational Leadership,* May 1983, 4-8.

Burney, G. M. Logical reasoning test. In R. B. Sund (Ed.), *Piaget for Educators*. Columbus, Ohio: Charles E. Merrill Publishing Company, 1976, 1975, 165-173.

Carter, R. The beginner's guide to logo. *Classroom Computer News*, April, 1983, 35-39.

Elkind, D. Adolescent thinking and the curriculum. *New York Education Quarterly*, Fall 1980, 18-24.

Eisner, E. The role of the arts in cognition and curriculum. *Phi Delta Kappan*, 1981, *63*(1), 48-53.

Epstein, H. Phrenoblysis: special brain and mind growth periods. *Developmental Psychobiology*, 1974, *3*, 207-224.

Epstein, H. Growth spurts during brain development: implications for educational policy. In J. Chall and A. Mirsky (Eds.), *Education and the brain*, seventy-seventh yearbook of the national society for the study of education, II. Chicago: University of Chicago Press, 1978.

Epstein, H. Correlated brain and intelligence development in humans. In M. E. Hahn, D. Jensen & B. Dudek (Eds.), *Development and evolution of brain size*, New York: Academic Press, 1979.

Epstein, H. Learning to learn: matching instructional levels. *The Principal*, May, 1981, 25-30.

Gardner, D. P. (Chairman). A nation at risk. (Report of the National Commission on Excellence in Education, U. S. Department of Education, Stock No. 065-000-00177-2). Washington, D. C.: U. S. Government Printing Office, 1983.

Gazzaniga, M. Cerebral dominance viewed as a decision system. In S. Dimons and J. Beaumont (Eds.), *Hemispheric functions in the human brain*. London: Halstead Press, 1974.

Glassner, B. Preliminary report: Hemispheric relationships in composing. *Journal of Education*, Spring 1980, *162*, 74-95.

Haglund, E. A closer look at the brain as related to teachers and learners. *Peabody Journal of Education*, 1981, *58*(4), 225-235.

Hart, L. *How the brain works: A new understanding of human learning, emotion, and thinking*. New York: Basic Books, 1975.

Hart, L. Brain-compatible education. In *Student learning styles and brain behavior*. Reston, VA: National Association of Secondary School Principals, 1982.

Hopkins, L. T. *Integration: its meaning and application*. New York: Appleton-Century-Crofts, 1937.

Kinsbourne, M., & Hiscock, M. Cerebral lateralization and cognitive development. In J. Chall and A. Mirsky (Eds.), *Education and the brain*, seventy-seventh yearbook of the national society for the study of education, II. Chicago: University of Chicago Press, 1978.

Krug, E. *Curriculum planning* (rev. ed.). New York: Harper & Bros. 1957.

Lawson, A. The development and validation of a classroom test of formal operations. *Journal of Research in Science Teaching*, 1978, *15*, 11-24.

Levin, J. What have we learned about maximizing what children learn? In J. Levin & V. Allen (Eds.), *Cognitive learning in children: Theories and strategies*. New York: Academic Press, Inc., 1976.

Levy, J. Children think with whole brains: Myth and reality. In *Student learning styles and brain behavior*. Reston, VA: National Association of Secondary School Principals, 1982.

Lough, T. Discovery of learning with the classroom's newest pet. *Electronic Learning*, March, 1983a, 49-53.

Lough, T. Exploring new horizons with logo. *Electronic Learning*. April, 1983b, 71-74.

McCarthy, B. *The 4 mat system: teaching to learning styles using left/right mode techniques*. Oak Brook, IL: Excell, 1982.

Ojemann, G., as reported in Begley, S., Carey, J., & Sawhill, R. How the brain works. *Newsweek*, February 7, 1983, 40-47.

Reynolds, C. R. Neorological assessment in education: a caution. *Journal of research and development in education,* Spring, 1982, 76-79.

Riegel, T., Jr. A lateralization study with high school students and unanswered questions underlying the emerging left-right model. Paper presented at the Conference on the Relationship of Cerebral Lateralization in Education, Atlanta, GA, April 20, 1979.

Sherman, V. In Brain-mid bulletin, Los Angeles, CA. (Reprinted in B. Stalyean (Ed.), *Together: Notes on humanistic education,* Association for Humanistic Psychology, June 1979, 9.)

Sinatra, R. Brain research sheds light on language learning. *Educational Leadership,* May 1983, 9-12.

Strahan, D. Problem solving strategies of early adolescent readers: A naturalistic protocol analysis. *Reading Improvement,* 1982, *19*(3), 183-194.

Toepfer, C., Jr. *Brain growth periodization: curricular implications for nursery through grade 12 learning.* Paper presented to the annual meeting of the Association for Supervision and Curriculum Development, St. Louis, Missouri, March, 1981 (ERIC Document, Reproduction Service No. ED 204 835 EA 013 727.)

Toepfer, C. F., Jr. Curriculum design and neuropsychological development. *Journal of research and development in education,* Spring, 1982, 1-11.

Torrance, E. P., Reynolds, C. R., Riegel, T., & Ball, O. E. Your style of learning and thinking, forms a and b: preliminary norms, abbreviated technical notes, scoring keys and selected references. *Gifted Child Quarterly,* 1977, *21,* 563-573.

SELECTED READINGS

Books

THE HUMAN BRAIN, Edited by M. C. Wittrock. Englewood Cliffs: Prentice Hall, 1977, 182 pages.

Eminent neurobiologists, neurosurgeons, psychologists, psychiatrists, and educational psychologists have written a book about recent research on the structure and function of the brain for teachers, school administrators, guidance counselors, psychologists, and lay people. For this readership, they have focused on the fundamental processes and structure of the human brain, the hemispheric process, and the educational implications. The contents are further substantiated with illustrations, charts, and a glossary. It is recommended as a desk copy. The references are as timely today as when it was published.

THE BRAIN: THE LAST FRONTIER, by Richard Restak. New York: Warner Books, 1979, 445 pages.

Richard Restak, a neurologist, substantiates a rationale for following the functional organization approach for studying the brain as used by psychobiologists instead of the behavioral approach as used by behavioral psychologists. The former approach is more complex and offers a wider latitude for future studies. The latter approach is more simplistic but only allows limited opportunities for future explorations. Restak explains how the working brain through the evolutionary process inherits unlearned, preprogrammed sets of behavior such as perception, intuition, establishing territorial rights, and many other behaviors. He further explains how the development of the working brain is influenced by contemporary parent-child relationships, child-rearing patterns, and health conditions including nutritional influences, social attitudes, cultural patterns, and environmental conditions. Technological advances, microcircuitry, and holography will lead to further explorations on the functional processes. In conclusion, Restak states that by the turn-of-the century, "our approach to the brain will again be radically different from our present orientation." The use of non-scientific language and everyday analogies makes this book comprehensive but easy to read.

UNDERSTANDING THE ALPHA CHILD AT HOME AND SCHOOL: LEFT AND RIGHT HEMISPHERIC FUNCTION IN RELATION TO PERSONALITY AND LEARNING, by Jack Fadely and Virginia Hosler. Springfield, Illinois: Thomas, 1979, 256 pages.

The authors describe children whose strengths lie in the gestalt, nonverbal capabilities of the right cerebral hemisphere and the problems they face in our left hemisphere-oriented schools. They believe that this "alpha" child is often mislabeled as hyperactive, learning disabled, or mentally disabled.

Their review of cerebral laterality and organization is both readable and accurate. The inclusion of rating scales designed to identify the alpha child can be used by anyone interested in investigating what appears to be an emerging major learning style element.

STUDENT LEARNING STYLES. Reston, Va.: National Association of Secondary School Principals, 1979.

A newly released unique compendium of articles authored by leaders in the field of learning styles makes this an important contribution to the literature on the teaching-learning process. *Student Learning Styles* successfully integrates the various forces which have directly and indirectly shaped the theory and practice of learning styles during the past fifteen years.

The book addresses teachers, administrators, counselors, and psychologists. Practical, field-tested techniques for diagnosing the learning styles of pupils for the purposes of individualizing instruction, creating appropriate classroom environments, and interviewing or counseling are amply illustrated. The cognitive, affective, physiological and psychological parameters of learning style are fully articulated. In addition, learning style assessment instruments are identified along with exciting, new research on brain hemisphere functions.

The wealth of insights assembled in this book should prove to be most useful to the practitioner as well as the researcher interested in identifying, comprehending, and responding to the variety of learning styles pupils carry with them.

DRAWING ON THE RIGHT SIDE OF THE BRAIN: A COURSE IN ENHANCING CREATIVITY AND ARTISTIC CONFIDENCE, by Betty Edwards. Los Angeles: J. P. Tarcher, Inc., 1979.

Applying recent discoveries on left and right brain hemisphere learning to the teaching of drawing skills, Edwards presents a set of basic exercises, designed to release creative potential and tap into the spatial, intuitive, and holistic modes of the right side of the brain. She verifies the importance of identifying a person's learning style and changing the educational environment from one that is mainly verbal, symbolic, abstract, and analytical to accommodate visual, nonverbal, and concrete modes as well. She advocates that, ultimately, the goal of education must be to develop both hemispheres of the brain, since both modes are necessary for full human functioning and creativity. Hence *Drawing on the Right Side of the Brain* is an important new dimension for all who seek to maximize learning potentials.

HUMAN BRAIN AND HUMAN LEARNING, by Leslie A. Hart. New York: Longman, 1983, 195 pages.

Leslie A. Hart is a generalist, a consultant, and a journalist who has devoted much of his career to studying the human brain. From these studies he has written many articles and books specifically geared toward educators. In this most recent book, the Proster theory is the central theme. Most of the chapters provide the background information for a theory he has developed over the past several years. It is based on research findings from ethology, anthropology, archeology, evolutionary science, neuroscience, computer science, cognitive psychology, behavioral psychology, education, and primate studies. The theory is based on two fundamental components; the brain is an "amazingly subtle and sensitive *pattern-detecting* apparatus" of which the development of pattern-detection is dependent on random and unorganized *input;* the extraction of patterns leads to the development of *programs* that are constantly being used, consciously and subconsciously, by the process of evaluation, selection, and implementation. Thus a proster may be defined as *a collection of stored programs, related to a particular pattern, which can be used as alternatives.* He recommends that this theory be a "replacement" for out-moded educational school systems as it can be applied to teaching, and to classroom settings. In conclusion, he states twelve broad-range benefits of this theory. Other distinguishing features include excellent analogies, guidelines and in-depth notes at the end of each chapter, a glossary, and an annotated bibliography.

PERSPECTIVES ON COGNITIVE SCIENCE, by Donald A. Norman. Norwood, N.J.: Ablex Publishing Corp./Hillsdale, N.J.: Lawrence Erlbaum Associates, 1981, 295 pages.

Donald Norman is a psychologist who was instrumental in organizing a conference that would mark the birth of *Cognitive Science*. The book is a collection of papers presented at that conference which address the need to merge into a new field since developments within the present day society do not fit into existing disciplines. The central theme of the book is based on the role of computation and symbol manipulation in cognition. "The human and the computer share the ability to create, manipulate, and process abstract symbols." Also in the book, the contributors discuss the way in which environment, society, cultures, and biology influence symbol manipulation. Underlying and related to these two themes are concerns about the evolution of the brain, constraints of symbol processing systems, concerns about memory, concerns about how humans reason, the role of intention, and language as it reflects man's internal, mental models. In conclusion, Norman discusses twelve issues that are key to the development, emotion, interaction, language, learning, memory, perception, performance, skill, and thought. This book is of value to educators because much that was discussed in the content of *A Child's Brain: The Impact of Advanced Research on Cognitive and Social Behaviors* is based on the research findings of these disciplines. In the future, it is likely teaching theories and teaching models will be strongly influenced by cognitive scientists.

OTHER BOOKS

Beadle, M. *A child's brain.* Garden City, N.Y.: Doubleday Anchor, 1971.

Blakemore, C. *Mechanics of the mind.* New York: Cambridge University Press, 1977.

Hart, L. *How the brain works.* New York, Basic Books, 1975.

Hart, L. *Teaching for learnings.* In press.

Hunt, M. *The Universe within.* New York: Simon & Schuster, 1982.

Kaufman, L. *Perception.* New York: Oxford University Press, 1979.

Sagan, C. *The dragons of eden.* New York: Random House, 1977.

Smith, F. *Comprehension and learnings.* New York: Holt, Rinehart and Winston, 1975.

The Diagram Group. *The brain: A user's manual.* New York: Perigee, G. P. Putnam's Sons, 1982.

Young. J. *Programs of the brain.* New York: Oxford University Press, 1978.

JOURNAL ARTICLES

Hart, L. Don't teach them; Help them learn. *Learning,* March 1981.

Hart, L. Classrooms are killing learning. *Principal,* May 1981.

Hart, L. The incredible brain: How does it solve problems? *Bulletin* National Association of Secondary School Principals, January 1983.

Hart, L. A quick tour of the brain. *The School Administrator,* January 1983.

DOCUMENTS AND JOURNAL ARTICLES FROM THE ERIC *DATABASE OR/FROM* ERIC

ASSESSMENT OF HEMISPHERIC DOMINANCE FOR LANGUAGE AT THREE AGES, by Deborah Walker Tagano. (1982, 15p., ED 220 177).

A study of children ages 4, 7, and 10 was conducted to assess the development of hemispheric dominance for language function and to determine whether age predicts hemispheric dominance. Dichotic listening-task performances suggested that differences between right- and left-hemisphere scores decreased with children's age. Given the traditional emphasis on left-hemisphere learning in schools, more right-brain experiences are recommended for young children.

AUDITORY ATTENDING SKILLS, by Sarah S. Van Camp. (1980, 17p., ED 188 760).

In order to tap left-hemisphere functioning, investigators told a story incorporating approximately 77 plot details to 42 preschool and kindergarten children. Measures of children's retellings, handedness, and eye dominance were obtained; results of individual profile analyses indicated that 50 percent of the children had major discrepancies in hemispheric functioning, suggesting clear differences in "learning style."

BRAIN LATERALIZATION IN INFANCY: IMPLICATIONS FOR DEVELOPMENT, by Rick Brooks. (1979, 14p., ED 183 243).

Briefly described are sources of evidence for hemispheric asymmetry in infants: the physical structure of the brain, hand preference, and responses to visual and auditory stimuli. It is suggested that, although little is known about the relationship between different types of stimuli and hemispheric activation, infants may benefit from a wide variety of left- and right-brain experiences.

CEREBRAL ASYMMETRY AND THE DEVELOPMENT OF INFANTILE AUTISM (Report No. 64), by Edward G. Blackstock. (1977, 29p., ED 146 749).

Examined in this discussion is the notion that, from birth, autistic children process information predominantly by strategies of the right-cerebral hemisphere and that they continue to be right-hemisphere processors throughout their lives. Two preliminary studies are cited in support of this idea, and implications of a new model for the diagnosis and treatment of autism are suggested.

EDUCATING THE OTHER HALF: IMPLICATIONS OF LEFT/RIGHT BRAIN RESEARCH, by Ronald L. Rubenner. (1982, 42p., ED 224 268).

Examines left/right brain research as it relates to learning and teaching styles, especially concerning children with special needs.

Methods for educational assessment of learning styles are reviewed, and steps toward dealing with the "whole child" are illuminated. Following discussion of implications of research for education, appendices present 35 activities to stimulate integrated left/right brain processes in children.

STUDENT LEARNING STYLES AND BRAIN BEHAVIOR: PROGRAMS, INSTRUMENTATION, RESEARCH. (1982, 235p., ED 227 565—document available on microfiche only.)

Collects 32 papers presented at a national conference sponsored by the Learning Styles Network of the National Association of Secondary School Principals. Specifically, papers offer comment on attempts to implement learning-styles analysis and diagnostic-prescriptive education in schools and classrooms, student learning-style assessment models and related research, in brain behavior research and applications, and next steps for study. Appendices include a student learning-styles model, an annotated bibliography, and information about the Network.

JOURNAL ARTICLES

BLACK-WHITE IQ DISCREPANCIES MAY BE RELATED TO DIFFERENCES IN HEMISPHERICITY, by Cecil R. Reynolds and others. *Contemporary Educational Psychology, 6*(2), 1981, 180-184.

The Weschler Preschool and Primary Scale of Intelligence and the McCarthy Scales subtests were ranked according to relative reliance on left-cerebral hemisphere function. Results suggested that IQ discrepancies between blacks and whites may be partially explained by differences in hemisphericity.

BRAIN LATERALIZATION: IMPLICATIONS FOR INFANT STIMULATION AND DEVELOPMENT, by Richard L. Brooks and John E. Obrzut. *Young Children, 36*(3), 9-16.

Discussed in this article are the implications of lateral dominance for infant stimulation and development. Also addressed are the concerns of parents and teachers as they relate to experiences for infants.

CEREBRAL ASYMMETRY AND HEMISPHERIC SPECIAL-
ISATION: SOME IMPLICATIONS OF SEX DIFFERENCES, by
Corinne Hutt. *International Journal of Behavioral Development,*
1979, 2(1), 73-86.

The author selectively reviews evidence for the cerebral organization and hemispheric specialization of language and visuospatial
function. Three theoretical models of cerebral organization are outlined, and some neuropsychological and educational implications
of sex differences in hemispheric specialization are considered.

A COMPARISON OF HEMISPHERIC PREFERENCE BE-
TWEEN HIGH-ABILITY AND LOW-ABILITY ELEMENTARY
CHILDREN, by Maureen Shannon and Dale R. Rice. *Educational
Research Quarterly,* 1982, 7(3), 7-15.

Hemispheric preferences of 70 high- and low-ability right-
handed elementary school children were investigated. Data obtained on the "Your Style of Learning and Thinking" instrument
revealed that the high-ability group had a greater preference for integrated functioning responses.

LATERAL PREFERENCE BEHAVIORS IN PRESCHOOL
CHILDREN AND YOUNG ADULTS, by Stanley Coren and others. *Child Development, 52*(2), 1981, 443-50.

Behavioral manifestations of hand, eye, foot, and ear preference
were studied in a sample of 384 children 3, 4, and 5 years of age.
When children's preferences were compared with those of a group
of 171 high-school students, results indicated that some aspects of
lateral preference behavior are influenced by age-related variables.

LATERALITY AND DIRECTIONAL PREFERENCES IN PRE-
SCHOOL CHILDREN, by Leslie E. Tan. *Perceptual and Motor
Skills,* 1982, 55(3), 863-70.

Three drawing tests provided for an assessment of left- or right-
handed 4-year-olds' directional preference for horizontal hand
movements. Directionality for more complex perceptual-motor
tasks was found to have a basis different from that of directionality
for simple tasks.

The ERIC documents and journal articles summarized above
were selected from a search of the Educational Resources Informa-

tion Center (ERIC) database. ERIC, the Education Resources Information Center, is funded by the National Institute of Education, U.S. Department of Education. Within the ERIC system are 16 separate clearinghouses, each responsible for collecting and disseminating information on a specific subject area in education. The ERIC Clearinghouse on Elementary and Early Childhood Education (ERIC/EECE) deals with information relating to the education and development of children from birth through age 12.

ERIC DOCUMENTS (those with ED numbers) are cited as abstracted in the monthly index *Resources in Education (RIE)*. The majority of these documents may be read on microfiche at the many libraries and information service agencies housing ERIC microfiche collections. In addition, most are available on microfiche or in paper copy from the ERIC Document Reproduction Service, P.O. Box 190, Arlington, VA 22210. Since prices are subject to change, please contact ERIC/EECE or consult the most recent issue of *RIE* for ordering information.

JOURNAL ARTICLES are cited and annotated in the monthly publication *Current Index to Journals in Education (CIJE)*. These articles may be read in periodicals obtained in libraries or through subscription. Selected article reprints are available from University Microfilms International, Article Reprint Department, 300 N. Zeeb Road, Ann Arbor, MI 48106. Please contact ERIC/EECE or see the most recent issue of *CIJE* for UMI ordering details.